METABOLIC SYNDROME ELIMINATION DIET

Transform Your Health, Lose Weight, Improve Insulin Sensitivity, and Prevent Type 2 Diabetes

Joe Miller, RD

COPYRIGHT PAGE

Table of Contents

COPYRIGHT PAGE..2

Table of Contents..3

INTRODUCTION 1

WHAT YOU SHOULD UNDERSTAND ABOUT METABOLIC SYNDROME 6

Who usually ends up with Metabolic Syndrome?..9

What kind of health issues might I face if I end up with metabolic syndrome?............................12

WHAT LEADS TO METABOLIC SYNDROME? 18

Understanding When to Seek Medical Help ..22

SIGNS AND CLUES THAT YOU MIGHT BE EXPERIENCING METABOLIC SYNDROME 24

How We Can Keep Metabolic Syndrome at Bay 29

DETECTING METABOLIC SYNDROME 35

How do we treat and handle Metabolic Syndrome? 39

What your doctor's approach should involve: 45

HEALTHY DISHES FOR METABOLIC SYNDROME 49

DELICIOUS MORNING DISH IDEAS FOR METABOLIC SYNDROME 50

Porridge 51

Instant Pot Steel-Cut Oats 53

Muesli 54

High-Protein Oatmeal for Athletes 56

Low-Fat Blueberry Bran Muffins 57

Quinoa Porridge 59

Apple Cinnamon Oatmeal 61

Reduced Fat French Toast 62

Refried Beans, Pico and Sunny Side Egg Breakfast Toast 64

Cocoa Cherry Protein Shake 65

Mixed Berry Smoothie 66

Banana Oat Smoothie 68

Tropical Protein Smoothie 69

Avocado & Egg Toast 70

Easy Quinoa Porridge With Golden Milk 72

Coconut Gluten-Free Pancakes with Berry Syrup 75

Millet Breakfast Porridge 77

Overnight Oatmeal With Dried Cherries 80

Tahini & Apple Oatmeal 82

Vanilla Chia Pudding 83

DELICIOUS LUNCH IDEAS FOR METABOLIC SYNDROME......86

Lentil Salad With Cumin & Orange Vinaigrette 86

Chicken Sancocho......91

Baked Falafel 97

Brussels Sprout Pita Pizza......99

Eggplant Pita Pizza 101

Sweet Potato Chickpea Bowl 104

Vegetarian Shepherd's Pie 108

Curried Chickpea Patties 111

Granola-Stuffed Winter Squash 114

Kale & Lemon Barlotto 118

Moroccan Vegetable Stew 120

Refried Beans, Pico and Sunny Side Egg Breakfast Toast......125

Citrus Quinoa Avocado Salad 126

Cocoa Cherry Protein Shake 129

Avocado & Egg Toast 130

Easy Quinoa Porridge With Golden Milk 131

Chickpea Salad Sandwich 134

Honey Mustard Chicken Salad 137

Chicken Enchilada-Stuffed Zucchini Boats ...141

Ham & Cheese Chicken Rollups 144

Portobello Fajita Bowl Meal Prep 148

Tofu Stir Fry 153

Sheet Tray Fajitas Rice Bowl 156

Eggplant Parmesan Boats 159

Lentil & Roasted Vegetable Salad 162

Zucchini "Enchiladas" 166

Cauliflower Walnut Burritos 169

Healthier Veggie Fried Rice............................173

TASTY DINNERTIME DISHES FOR METABOLIC
SYNDROME..178

Vegan Lasagna Soup....................................178

Whole Wheat Pasta With Lemon Kale Chicken
....181

Fajita Pasta Bake 184

Loaded Baked Potato Soup..........................188

Penne Alla Vodka Pasta 191

Chorizo Tomato Rotini Pasta........................194

Spinach Mushroom Pesto Spaghetti.............196

Caprese Spaghetti Squash...........................198

Crunchy Avocado Tuna Wraps 202

Tomato Basil Sausage Spaghetti 204

One-Pan Chicken And Broccoli Stir Fry 206

Slow Cooker Balsamic Chicken....................209

Instant Pot Butter Chicken 211

Chickpea Sweet Potato Stew 216

Caprese Spaghetti Squash................220

Crunchy Avocado Tuna Wraps 224

Roasted Eggplant Curry...................226

Parchment Teriyaki Salmon...........230

Easy Salmon Dinner.........................233

Sausage, Spinach, Tomato Rigatoni...............236

Sesame Peanut Noodles 240

SWEET TREATS FOR METABOLIC SYNDROME
....243

Strawberry Banana Chia Seed Pudding.........243

Easiest Banana-cocoa Ice Cream 245

Strawberry Chocolate Mousse 247

Frozen Banana Ice Cream 249

Iced Oatmeal Cookies 251

Apple Pie (Macerated).................................255

Banana Berry Fruit Salad 259

Kiwi Sorbet...261

Vegan Apple Pie...262

Banana Bread Dip.......................................267

CONCLUSION 269

INTRODUCTION

Excess weight and obesity have been intricately linked with the development of a complex array of health issues known as metabolic syndrome, encompassing various vascular and metabolic diseases. Within the medical community, there's a consensus that this syndrome manifests through several key markers, including reduced insulin sensitivity, elevated blood sugar levels (hyperglycemia), abnormal lipid levels (dyslipidemia), particularly high triglycerides coupled with low HDL-cholesterol, abdominal obesity, and hypertension. Despite these recognized indicators, there isn't a universally accepted set of diagnostic criteria.

Metabolic syndrome represents a constellation of metabolic risk factors that significantly elevate the likelihood of developing severe conditions such as cancer, heart disease, dementia, and Type 2 diabetes. Moreover, individuals with metabolic syndrome often experience chronic, low-grade systemic inflammation, further predisposing them to serious consequences like increased susceptibility to infections such as the flu and COVID-19. A diagnosis of metabolic syndrome serves as a red flag indicating malfunctioning metabolic health, signifying the body's compromised ability to efficiently utilize and process nutrients and energy from food. Without intervention, the risks to health only escalate.

Alarming statistics underscore the pervasive nature of this syndrome, with approximately 50%

of Americans over 60 years old diagnosed with metabolic syndrome between 2011 and 2016. What's more concerning is the rising prevalence among adolescents, paralleling the uptrend in rates of overweight and obesity. Often, individuals receive various diagnoses preceding a diagnosis of metabolic syndrome, such as hypertension or elevated blood sugar levels, which collectively point to underlying metabolic dysfunction.

A diagnosis of metabolic syndrome signifies a breakdown in a person's metabolic equilibrium, highlighting the urgency for lifestyle modifications to mitigate disease risks. For healthcare providers, this diagnosis serves as a roadmap, prompting further assessment for additional risk factors and initiating tailored treatment protocols.

Based on current estimates utilizing established criteria, metabolic syndrome affects a substantial proportion of middle-aged and elderly populations across European countries, increasing the risk for Type 2 diabetes and cardiovascular disease manifold and significantly impacting morbidity rates. Insulin resistance and abdominal obesity emerge as pivotal factors driving alterations in glucose and lipid metabolism, as well as vascular function, culminating in the development of Type 2 diabetes, atherosclerosis, and cardiovascular disease, even though the precise mechanisms remain incompletely understood.

The intricate interplay between metabolic syndrome, Type 2 diabetes, and cardiovascular disease, coupled with the challenge of stemming the rising tide of obesity, foreshadows an unsustainable burden on healthcare systems over the coming decades. To curb the proliferation of metabolic syndrome and alleviate the strain on healthcare resources, proactive measures are imperative. Recent research indicating the superiority of lifestyle interventions, including dietary modifications and increased physical activity, over pharmacological approaches in preventing Type 2 diabetes in high-risk individuals represents a pivotal advancement in this endeavor.

CHAPTER 1
WHAT YOU SHOULD UNDERSTAND ABOUT METABOLIC SYNDROME

Metabolic syndrome, a cluster of heart disease risk factors, presents a significant health concern as it heightens one's susceptibility to conditions like diabetes, heart disease, and stroke. This multifaceted health issue, often dubbed Syndrome X, insulin resistance syndrome, or dysmetabolic syndrome, is a complex interplay of various physiological factors that culminate in detrimental health outcomes.

Statistics from a comprehensive national health survey reveal that metabolic syndrome affects more than one in five Americans, underscoring its pervasive impact on public health. Moreover, the prevalence of this syndrome escalates with age, with over 40% of individuals in their 60s and 70s experiencing its effects.

Metabolic syndrome isn't merely a standalone condition; rather, it's a constellation of interconnected health markers, including elevated blood pressure, high blood sugar levels, abnormal cholesterol levels, and excess abdominal fat. This confluence of factors not only increases the risk of cardiovascular ailments but also significantly raises the likelihood of developing type 2 diabetes.

Understanding the dynamics of metabolic syndrome involves recognizing its intricate relationship with lifestyle factors such as poor diet, sedentary habits, and obesity. These lifestyle choices can exacerbate the underlying metabolic dysregulation, perpetuating a cycle of deteriorating health outcomes.

Addressing metabolic syndrome requires a multifaceted approach encompassing lifestyle modifications, dietary interventions, regular physical activity, and, in some cases, pharmacological interventions. By adopting proactive measures to manage metabolic risk factors, individuals can mitigate their susceptibility to debilitating health conditions associated with this syndrome.

Metabolic syndrome poses a considerable public health challenge, necessitating comprehensive strategies to curb its prevalence and mitigate its adverse health consequences across diverse demographic groups.

Who usually ends up with Metabolic Syndrome?

Metabolic syndrome, a multifaceted health condition characterized by a combination of central obesity, insulin resistance, elevated blood pressure, and abnormal lipid levels, presents a substantial risk to individuals' overall well-being. Specifically, those who carry excess fat around their waist and abdomen are more susceptible to this syndrome, as are individuals with a diagnosis of diabetes mellitus or a strong family history of the disease.

Moreover, certain clinical symptoms indicative of insulin resistance, such as skin tags or acanthosis nigricans (a darkening of the skin typically seen on the back of the neck), further heighten the risk of developing metabolic syndrome. Additionally, individuals from specific ethnic backgrounds may face an increased predisposition to this syndrome, highlighting the complex interplay between genetic and environmental factors in its development.

Furthermore, it's essential to recognize that the likelihood of acquiring metabolic syndrome rises with age, underscoring the importance of early detection and proactive management strategies. As individuals progress through life stages, physiological changes and lifestyle factors can exacerbate the underlying metabolic disturbances associated with this condition, necessitating ongoing monitoring and intervention to reduce the risk of complications such as cardiovascular disease and type 2 diabetes.

Metabolic syndrome represents a significant health concern with diverse contributing factors, including genetic predisposition, lifestyle choices, and demographic variables. Addressing these complexities requires a comprehensive approach that integrates medical management, behavioral modifications, and community-based interventions to promote optimal health outcomes and mitigate the long-term consequences of metabolic dysfunction.

What kind of health issues might I face if I end up with metabolic syndrome?

Elevated levels of insulin and glucose in the body can precipitate a cascade of detrimental effects, each of which poses a significant threat to overall health and wellbeing. These effects extend across various bodily systems, manifesting in several ways:

Firstly, heightened insulin and glucose levels contribute to the injury and dysfunction of the lining of coronary arteries and other vital arteries.

This damage serves as a pivotal precursor to the onset of severe cardiovascular conditions such as heart disease or stroke, both of which can have profound and potentially life-threatening implications.

Furthermore, the metabolic imbalance associated with elevated insulin and glucose levels can impair the kidneys' ability to regulate salt excretion effectively. This impairment can lead to the development of hypertension, further escalating the risk of cardiovascular complications including heart disease and stroke.

Moreover, an increase in triglyceride levels, a type of fat found in the blood, is closely linked with elevated insulin and glucose levels. Elevated triglycerides significantly heighten the risk of developing cardiovascular diseases, thereby compounding the already substantial dangers posed by metabolic dysregulation.

Additionally, elevated insulin and glucose levels increase the likelihood of blood clot formation within the circulatory system. These blood clots can obstruct arteries, impeding the flow of blood to vital organs such as the heart and brain, consequently precipitating heart attacks or strokes with potentially devastating consequences.

Moreover, a decrease in insulin production, often associated with prolonged periods of elevated insulin and glucose levels, can serve as an early warning sign for the onset of type 2 diabetes. This chronic metabolic disorder significantly amplifies the risk of experiencing cardiovascular events such as heart attacks and strokes, exacerbating the already precarious state of cardiovascular health.

Moreover, uncontrolled diabetes can also lead to a myriad of other complications affecting various bodily systems. Eye, nerve, and renal complications are commonly observed consequences of poorly managed diabetes, further underscoring the multifaceted risks associated with metabolic dysregulation.

Furthermore, there exists a correlation between elevated insulin and glucose levels and liver inflammation, particularly in the form of non-alcoholic steatohepatitis (NASH), a type of fatty liver disease. If left untreated, NASH can progress to more severe liver conditions such as cirrhosis and liver failure, underscoring the critical importance of addressing metabolic dysregulation to mitigate the risk of debilitating liver complications.

The ramifications of elevated insulin and glucose levels extend far beyond mere metabolic dysregulation, encompassing a broad spectrum of cardiovascular, metabolic, and hepatic complications, each of which underscores the imperative of proactive management and intervention to safeguard against potentially catastrophic health outcomes.

CHAPTER 2
WHAT LEADS TO METABOLIC SYNDROME?

It's possible that within your genetic makeup lies a susceptibility to metabolic syndrome, a cluster of conditions including increased blood pressure, high blood sugar, excess body fat around the waist, and abnormal cholesterol or triglyceride levels. While genetics can play a role, for most individuals, the primary culprits behind the development of overweight, obesity (particularly abdominal or visceral fat), and consequently, metabolic syndrome, are rooted in lifestyle factors.

Let's delve into the intricate web of causality. One significant player in this narrative is gut dysbiosis, an imbalance between beneficial and harmful bacteria in your digestive system. This delicate balance can be disrupted by various factors, such as poor dietary choices lacking in fiber-rich plant foods, overuse of antibiotics, chronic stress, among others. When the scales tip towards harmful bacteria, particularly gram-negative ones, they release endotoxins (lipopolysaccharides or LPS) into your system. These endotoxins trigger an inflammatory response, prompting the release of pro-inflammatory cytokines, the molecular messengers orchestrating communication between your cells.

However, at the heart of metabolic syndrome lies insulin resistance, a condition where your body's cells become less responsive to the effects of insulin, leading to elevated blood sugar levels.

This insulin resistance sets off a cascade of detrimental effects, including further inflammation and oxidative stress, accelerating damage to the liver and blood vessels. Endothelial dysfunction, a hallmark of metabolic syndrome, is characterized by impaired functioning of the endothelium, the inner lining of blood vessels. This dysfunction not only paves the way for coronary artery disease but also exacerbates the inflammatory milieu within the body.

Moreover, when abdominal fat enters the equation, it acts as a potent fuel for the pro-inflammatory cycle. Excess visceral adipose tissue secretes inflammatory cytokines and adipokines, further fueling systemic inflammation and insulin resistance. This vicious cycle culminates in the development of non-alcoholic fatty liver disease

(NAFLD) and exacerbates the metabolic dysregulation characteristic of metabolic syndrome.

Thus, while genetic predispositions may set the stage, it is the interplay of lifestyle factors, gut health, insulin resistance, and inflammatory processes that ultimately drive the development and progression of metabolic syndrome. Addressing these underlying factors through targeted interventions aimed at improving dietary habits, reducing stress, and promoting physical activity is paramount in managing and preventing metabolic syndrome and its associated complications.

Understanding When to Seek Medical Help

If you find yourself struggling to rectify the metabolic imbalances induced by metabolic syndrome through adjustments in your dietary intake and exercise regimen alone, it may be time to consider medical intervention. Delving deeper into the nuances of managing your metabolic disorders through a holistic approach involving nutrition, physical activity, and medication warrants a conversation with your primary healthcare practitioner.

Your doctor possesses the expertise to guide you through addressing and managing your metabolic challenges utilizing what can be termed as an "ABCDE approach," which encompasses a thorough consideration of your pre-existing medical conditions. This approach ensures that all facets of your metabolic abnormalities are carefully attended to with tailored dietary modifications, suitable physical activities, and appropriate medications. By engaging in this comprehensive strategy, you pave the way towards fostering optimal metabolic health under the professional guidance of healthcare experts.

CHAPTER 3
SIGNS AND CLUES THAT YOU MIGHT BE EXPERIENCING METABOLIC SYNDROME

The prevalence of metabolic syndrome, a multifaceted health concern, is escalating at an alarming rate globally. Currently, approximately a quarter of the world's population is affected, with the incidence steadily climbing. Particularly noteworthy is the situation in the United States, where more than a third of the population grapples with this condition.

Metabolic syndrome, although not a standalone disease, constitutes a cluster of five interrelated symptoms that significantly elevate the risk of developing a spectrum of chronic health issues.

These encompass diabetes, cardiovascular ailments, kidney complications, strokes, and various other metabolic irregularities.

Unhealthy dietary habits, sedentary lifestyles, and inadequate physical activity are recognized as primary contributors to the onset of metabolic syndrome. Once diagnosed, this syndrome tends to deteriorate over time and, if left unaddressed, can lead to persistent and potentially fatal metabolic dysfunctions. Moreover, the presence of one metabolic syndrome component can exacerbate others, heightening the individual's susceptibility to a constellation of health challenges.

For instance, individuals diagnosed with diabetes are up to five times more likely to experience cardiovascular complications. Recognizing the warning signs or risk factors associated with metabolic syndrome is crucial for early intervention and management.

Elevated blood sugar levels represent a pivotal indicator, with fasting blood sugar levels exceeding 100 mg/dL signaling a pre-diabetic state. Family history of Type-2 diabetes and gestational diabetes further compounds the risk.

Another hallmark of metabolic syndrome is elevated blood pressure, often dubbed the "Silent Killer." This condition manifests when the force of blood against arterial walls exceeds healthy levels, imposing strain on the cardiovascular system and predisposing individuals to cardiac issues and related complications.

High triglyceride levels, stemming from excessive fat consumption, precipitate the deposition of fatty deposits within artery walls, escalating the risk of heart attacks and strokes.

Reduced levels of high-density lipoprotein (HDL), commonly referred to as "good cholesterol," compromise the body's ability to fend off cardiovascular threats, accentuating the accumulation of low-density lipoprotein (LDL) and narrowing arteries, thereby heightening the risk of heart attacks, strokes, and peripheral artery disease.

A significant waist circumference, indicative of central obesity or an "apple-shaped" body, augments the likelihood of metabolic syndrome. In males, waist sizes surpassing 40 inches and in females exceeding 35 inches are associated with heightened risks.

Metabolic syndrome represents a complex interplay of lifestyle factors and genetic predispositions, underscoring the importance of proactive measures such as dietary modifications, regular physical activity, and medical interventions to mitigate associated risks and promote long-term health and well-being.

How We Can Keep Metabolic Syndrome at Bay

Promoting and preserving metabolic health entails a multifaceted approach that delves deep into lifestyle adjustments, dietary choices, and overall well-being practices. Embarking on a journey toward metabolic equilibrium involves embracing a rich tapestry of behaviors and habits that foster vitality and longevity.

At the heart of this endeavor lies the indispensable significance of nurturing healthy eating habits. It beckons individuals to embark on a gastronomic adventure brimming with an abundance of nature's bounties: succulent fruits, hearty grains, pristine lean proteins, and verdant, crisp vegetables. It's a culinary symphony where the melody of health resonates through the inclusion of two servings of fruits and three servings of vegetables daily, alongside the incorporation of low-fat dairy products, fat-free or low-fat milk, and the wholesome embrace of whole-grain, high-fiber cereals.

Moreover, the pathway to metabolic nirvana is illuminated by the beacon of physical activity. Each day presents an opportunity to partake in the joyful dance of movement, where moderate to intense physical exertion for a minimum of thirty minutes, five days a week, becomes the norm.

Whether it's the rhythmic pound of running shoes on pavement, the leisurely stroll through nature's embrace, or the exuberant playfulness of recreational sports, the canvas of physical activity paints a picture of vitality and vigor.

Dietary modifications emerge as pivotal brushstrokes in this masterpiece of metabolic wellness. Saturated and trans fats, those nefarious adversaries to equilibrium, are relegated to the periphery as individuals opt for healthier alternatives, swapping solid fats for the liquid embrace of vegetable oils such as olive or canola. Carbohydrates, once perceived with trepidation, find redemption in the realm of whole grains, with brown rice and whole-grain bread emerging as stalwart allies. The dietary landscape is further enriched by the verdant bounty of dietary fiber found in whole grain products, legumes, fruits, and vegetables, while the consumption of poultry and red meat takes a backseat to the piscine delights of fish, devoid of skin and untouched by the searing kiss of frying.

In the realm of holistic well-being, the reduction of tension emerges as a cornerstone in the edifice of metabolic harmony. The deleterious effects of stress on metabolic equilibrium necessitate the adoption of practices that soothe the soul and calm the mind. Whether it's the graceful flow of yoga, the tranquil introspection of meditation, or the cleansing breaths of deep relaxation, the arsenal against stress becomes as diverse as it is potent.

Striving for one's desired weight constitutes yet another crucial facet in the mosaic of metabolic health. Shedding excess pounds becomes not merely a quest for aesthetic appeal but a journey toward enhanced vitality and well-being. Bid farewell to the siren call of "junk food," those tantalizing temptations laden with sodium, refined white flour, trans fats, added sugars, and solid fats. Instead, embrace a dietary paradigm characterized by wholesomeness and nutrition, where sugary beverages and calorie-laden treats find no sanctuary.

And amidst this tapestry of lifestyle modifications, one cannot overlook the insidious influence of smoking. A habit that not only imperils respiratory health but also casts a dark shadow over cardiovascular well-being, smoking stands as a formidable barrier on the path to metabolic equilibrium. Liberation from this pernicious habit not only heralds a brighter tomorrow but also serves as a testament to one's commitment to holistic health.

The journey toward metabolic wellness is not a solitary trek but a communal odyssey, where each step forward is buoyed by the collective wisdom of dietary mindfulness, physical activity, stress reduction, weight management, and the renunciation of deleterious habits. It's a journey that beckons all to embrace the transformative power of lifestyle modifications and emerge as stewards of their own metabolic destiny.

If you find yourself ticking off three or more of the following health markers, you might be dealing with metabolic syndrome, a cluster of conditions that can significantly impact your well-being:

1. Waist Circumference: Measure around your belly, and if it's at least 40 inches for men or 35 inches for women, you're on the radar for metabolic syndrome. This measurement isn't just about fitting into your favorite pair of jeans; it's a critical indicator of visceral fat accumulation, which is linked to metabolic dysfunction.

2. Blood Pressure: If your blood pressure consistently reads at 130/85 mm Hg or above, or if you're managing your blood pressure with medication, it's a red flag for metabolic syndrome. High blood pressure, especially when combined with other metabolic issues, can increase your risk of heart disease, stroke, and other complications.

3. Triglyceride Level: Keep an eye on your triglyceride levels. If they soar to 150 mg/dl or higher, it's another marker of metabolic syndrome. Elevated triglycerides are associated with insulin resistance and can contribute to cardiovascular problems.

4. Fasting Blood Sugar: A fasting blood sugar level above 100 mg/dl could indicate trouble, especially if you're not already managing it with medication. This suggests that your body might not be effectively regulating glucose, a hallmark feature of metabolic syndrome and diabetes.

5. Low HDL Cholesterol: HDL cholesterol, often dubbed the "good" cholesterol, plays a crucial role in heart health. For men, a level below 40 mg/dl, and for women, below 50 mg/dl, signals a risk factor for metabolic syndrome. Low HDL levels can impair the body's ability to remove LDL cholesterol from the bloodstream, increasing the risk of plaque buildup in arteries.

Understanding these interconnected factors is crucial because metabolic syndrome isn't just about a single measurement—it's about recognizing the intricate web of metabolic imbalances that can pave the way for serious health issues down the line. Taking proactive steps to address these markers through lifestyle changes, medication if necessary, and regular monitoring can help mitigate the risks associated with metabolic syndrome and promote better overall health and longevity.

How do we treat and handle Metabolic Syndrome?

Enhancing overall well-being and mitigating the onset of chronic conditions such as diabetes and heart disease stands as the paramount goal within the realm of traditional clinical intervention for individuals grappling with metabolic syndrome. This multifaceted approach encompasses a spectrum of strategies, each aimed at different facets of the condition:

First and foremost, pharmaceutical intervention takes precedence, constituting the frontline defense mechanism to regulate and manage the underlying conditions associated with metabolic syndrome. As articulated by Dr. Scher, it's not uncommon for individuals diagnosed with metabolic syndrome to find themselves reliant on an array of prescribed medications designed to tackle elevated cholesterol levels, hypertension, and aberrant blood sugar readings.

However, recognizing the inherent limitations of medication in addressing the root causes of the syndrome, a fundamental shift in lifestyle becomes imperative. While pharmaceuticals may serve to suppress symptomatic manifestations, they fall short in addressing the core etiological factors contributing to the condition's progression. Hence, embracing a holistic lifestyle overhaul emerges as a pivotal adjunct to clinical treatment. This paradigm shift underscores the significance of making sustainable lifestyle modifications to not only alleviate symptoms but also to rectify underlying metabolic dysregulation.

Indeed, the lifestyle modifications advocated for the prevention of metabolic syndrome align seamlessly with those recommended for its management and potential reversal. Embracing the principles of the four Cs - namely, dietary adjustments, regular exercise, stress management techniques, and prioritizing adequate sleep - lays the foundation for fostering metabolic health and thwarting the deleterious consequences of the syndrome.

Furthermore, vigilant monitoring of one's health status assumes paramount importance in navigating the labyrinthine landscape of metabolic syndrome management. Collaborating closely with a multidisciplinary team of healthcare professionals, including endocrinologists, cardiologists, and diabetes specialists, enables individuals to embark on a proactive journey towards optimal health outcomes. This collaborative approach entails devising a tailored surveillance regimen encompassing regular check-ups and screenings aimed at tracking key metabolic parameters.

In parallel with clinical assessments, empowering individuals with the tools and knowledge to engage in self-monitoring practices fosters a sense of agency and accountability in managing their health. Armed with readily accessible tools such as glucose meters, individuals can actively monitor critical metrics such as weight fluctuations, waist circumference, blood pressure readings, and blood glucose levels between clinical consultations. This proactive approach not only facilitates early detection of aberrations but also empowers individuals to make timely adjustments to their lifestyle and treatment regimens under the guidance of healthcare professionals.

Combating metabolic syndrome necessitates a multifaceted approach that transcends the confines of pharmacological intervention, encompassing comprehensive lifestyle modifications and vigilant health monitoring. By embracing this holistic framework, individuals can proactively navigate the complexities of metabolic syndrome management, thereby mitigating the risk of diabetes and heart disease while optimizing overall health and well-being.

What your doctor's approach should involve:

"Evaluating and treating cardiovascular disorders involves a comprehensive approach aimed at addressing various aspects of heart health and overall well-being. This multifaceted process encompasses a range of interventions and strategies tailored to individual needs.

Blood pressure management forms a crucial component of cardiovascular care, with an emphasis on monitoring and regulating blood pressure levels to reduce the risk of complications such as heart disease and stroke. This involves implementing lifestyle modifications, dietary changes, and, when necessary, medication to achieve optimal blood pressure control.

Cholesterol control is another vital aspect of cardiovascular health management, focusing on regulating cholesterol levels to mitigate the risk of atherosclerosis and related conditions. This entails dietary adjustments, exercise regimens, and pharmacological interventions aimed at achieving healthy lipid profiles.

Managing diabetes involves a holistic approach that integrates dietary management, regular physical activity, and medication to optimize blood sugar levels and prevent complications associated with diabetes mellitus. This comprehensive approach aims to empower individuals with diabetes to lead healthy lifestyles while effectively managing their condition.

Workout therapy plays a pivotal role in promoting cardiovascular health and overall wellness. Tailored exercise programs are designed to enhance cardiovascular fitness, strengthen the heart muscle, improve circulation, and manage weight, thereby reducing the risk of cardiovascular diseases and improving quality of life.

Evaluating and treating cardiovascular disorders encompasses a multidimensional approach that addresses various facets of heart health, including blood pressure management, cholesterol control, diabetes management, and the incorporation of workout therapy into daily routines. By adopting a comprehensive strategy that combines lifestyle modifications, dietary interventions, exercise regimens, and medical management, individuals can optimize their cardiovascular health and reduce the risk of cardiovascular diseases."

CHAPTER 5
HEALTHY DISHES FOR METABOLIC SYNDROME

DELICIOUS MORNING DISH IDEAS FOR METABOLIC SYNDROME

Maple and Brown Sugar Oatmeal

Things Needed

1 ½ cups water

¾ cup quick-cooking oats

1 tablespoon packed dark brown sugar

1 tablespoon maple syrup

Instructions

Bring water to a boil in a small pot. Add oats and cook, stirring, for 1 minute.

Remove from heat and stir in brown sugar and maple syrup. Let sit until desired thickness is reached, 2 to 3 minutes.

Porridge

Things Needed

2 ½ cups water

1 cup rolled oats

1 tablespoon white sugar

1 teaspoon salt

2 bananas, sliced

1 pinch ground cinnamon

½ cup cold milk (Optional)

Instructions

Combine water, oats, sugar, and salt in a saucepan. Add bananas and cinnamon. Bring to a boil, then reduce heat to low, and simmer until the liquid has been absorbed, stirring frequently.

Pour into bowls, and top each with a splash of cold milk.

Instant Pot Steel-Cut Oats

Things Needed

3 cups water

1 cup steel-cut oats

Instructions

Combine water and oats in a multi-functional pressure cooker (such as Instant Pot). Close and lock the lid. Select high pressure according to manufacturer's instructions; set timer for 3 minutes. Allow 10 to 15 minutes for pressure to build.

Release pressure using the natural-release method according to manufacturer's instructions, 10 to 40 minutes. Oats will thicken as they cool.

Tips

You can use soy milk or any nut milk in place of water.

Muesli

Things Needed

4 ½ cups rolled oats

1 cup raisins

½ cup toasted wheat germ

½ cup wheat bran

½ cup oat bran

½ cup chopped walnuts

¼ cup packed brown sugar

¼ cup raw sunflower seeds

Instructions

Combine oats, raisins, wheat germ, wheat bran, oat bran, walnuts, brown sugar, and sunflower seeds in a large bowl; mix well. Store muesli in an airtight container at room temperature for up to 2 months.

High-Protein Oatmeal for Athletes

Things Needed

1 cup oatmeal

1 scoop whey protein powder, or to taste

½ cup blueberries

2 tablespoons pumpkin seeds, or to taste

2 tablespoons raisins, or to taste

¼ cup skim milk, or as needed

Instructions

Combine oatmeal and protein powder in a microwave-safe bowl. Add blueberries, pumpkin seeds, and raisins. Add milk and heat in the microwave for about 1 minute. Stir before serving.

Low-Fat Blueberry Bran Muffins

Things Needed

1 ½ cups wheat bran

1 cup nonfat milk

½ cup unsweetened applesauce

1 egg

⅔ cup brown sugar

½ teaspoon vanilla extract

½ cup all-purpose flour

½ cup whole wheat flour

1 teaspoon baking soda

1 teaspoon baking powder

½ teaspoon salt

1 cup blueberries

Instructions

Preheat oven to 375 degrees F (190 degrees C). Grease muffin cups or use paper muffin liners. Mix together wheat bran and milk, and let stand for 10 minutes.

In a large bowl, mix together applesauce, egg, brown sugar, and vanilla. Beat in bran mixture.

Sift together all-purpose flour, whole wheat flour, baking soda, baking powder, and salt. Stir into bran mixture until just blended. Fold in blueberries. Scoop into muffin cups.

Bake in preheated oven for 15 to 20 minutes, or until tops spring back when lightly tapped.

Quinoa Porridge

Things Needed

½ cup quinoa

¼ teaspoon ground cinnamon

1 ½ cups almond milk

½ cup water

2 tablespoons brown sugar

1 teaspoon vanilla extract (Optional)

1 pinch salt

Instructions

Heat a saucepan over medium heat and measure in the quinoa. Season with cinnamon and cook until toasted, stirring frequently, about 3 minutes. Pour in the almond milk, water and vanilla and stir in the brown sugar and salt. Bring to a boil, then cook over low heat until the porridge is thick and grains are tender, about 25 minutes. Add more water if needed if the liquid has dried up before it finishes cooking. Stir occasionally, especially at the end, to prevent burning.

Apple Cinnamon Oatmeal

Things Needed

1 cup water

¼ cup apple juice

1 apple, cored and chopped

⅔ cup rolled oats

1 teaspoon ground cinnamon

1 cup milk

Instructions

Combine the water, apple juice, and apples in a saucepan. Bring to a boil over high heat, and stir in the rolled oats and cinnamon. Return to a boil, then reduce heat to low, and simmer until thick, about 3 minutes. Spoon into serving bowls, and pour milk over the servings.

Reduced Fat French Toast

Things Needed

½ cup egg substitute

⅔ cup skim milk

1 teaspoon vanilla extract

½ teaspoon ground cinnamon

6 slices reduced calorie white bread

Instructions

Beat together egg substitute, milk, vanilla and cinnamon. Dip bread slices in egg mixture until both sides are soaked.

Spray a skillet or frying pan with cooking spray and heat over medium high heat. Place bread slices into pan and cook until golden brown on both sides

Refried Beans, Pico and Sunny Side Egg Breakfast Toast

Things Needed

1 slice whole grain bread

2 Tbsp. refried beans, low sodium

1 Tbsp. pico de gallo

1 sunny side up egg

Instructions

Toast bread.

Warm beans on stovetop or in a microwave.

Cook egg sunny-side up.

Top all ingredients onto toast.

Cocoa Cherry Protein Shake

Things Needed

¾ cup whole milk

¼ cup Greek yogurt

½ cup frozen cherries

1 tbsp protein powder (see Chef Notes)

1 tbsp unsweetened cocoa powder

1 tbsp nut butter

1 tbsp flaxseed meal

½ cup ice

Instructions

Add all Things Needed to a high-speed blender and blend on high until smooth.

Serve immediately.

Mixed Berry Smoothie

Things Needed

1 cup frozen blackberries

½ cup frozen raspberries

½ avocado

½ cup Greek yogurt

1 cup whole milk

1 tbsp honey

½ tsp vanilla extract

Instructions

Add all ingredients to a high-speed blender and blend on high until smooth.

Serve immediately.

Banana Oat Smoothie

Things Needed

1 cup whole milk

1 tbsp nut butter

1 large banana

5-6 ice cubes

¼ cup rolled oats

½ tsp vanilla extract

¼ cup protein powder (see Chef Notes)

½ tsp cinnamon

Pinch of nutmeg

1 tbsp flaxseed meal

1 tbsp honey

Instructions

Add all Things Needed to a high-speed blender and blend on high until smooth.

Serve immediately.

Tropical Protein Smoothie

Things Needed

1 Navel orange

½ cup full fat coconut milk

¼ cup protein powder (see Chef Notes)

1 banana

½ avocado

½ cup ice

Instructions

Add all Things Needed to a high-speed blender and blend on high until smooth.

Serve immediately.

Avocado & Egg Toast

Things Needed

1/2 avocado, ripe

2 slices whole grain toast

Salt and pepper, to taste

Cayenne, to taste (optional)

Squeeze of lime (optional)

1 hard-boiled egg, sliced

Instructions

Scoop out the avocado flesh and spread it onto the toast by mashing it with the back of a fork.

Sprinkle salt, pepper, cayenne and squeeze of lime. Then layer hard-boiled egg slices on top of the avocado mash, and sprinkle with a little more salt and pepper.

Easy Quinoa Porridge With Golden Milk

Things Needed

1⅓ cups cooked quinoa (see Chef Tips)

1 cups 2% milk, or nondairy milk of choice

Pinch of sea salt

2 tablespoons cranberries

3 dates, pitted and chopped

1 teaspoon ginger root, freshly grated

½ teaspoon turmeric root, freshly grated (see Chef Tips)

1 cup apple, grated

⅓ cup fresh blueberries (optional)

2 tablespoons almonds, dry toasted and sliced

Plain Greek yogurt for serving (optional)

Instructions

In a small pot over medium-high heat, add the quinoa, milk, and a pinch of sea salt. Stir to mix. Add the cranberries, dates, grated ginger root, and turmeric. Stir again. Bring to a boil, cover, and turn the heat down to low. Cook for 5 to 8 minutes, stirring from time to time. For a thicker porridge, crack the lid.

Stir in the grated apple. Mix well. Cover and cook 2 to 3 minutes more. Add the blueberries and stir to mix. Cover, turn off the heat, and let sit for 2 to 3 minutes while you toast the nuts.

To dry toast the nuts: Heat a small heavy frying pan over medium-high heat. Add the nuts and cook, shaking until they are a light golden color — about 2 to 3 minutes. As soon as they are pale gold, turn off the heat, as there will be enough heat left to finish the toasting.

Serve the porridge in bowls with sprinkled with nuts and either with a dollop of plain Greek yogurt, if using, or with extra cold milk poured over it.

Coconut Gluten-Free Pancakes with Berry Syrup

Things Needed

2 cups mixed berries

⅓ cup brown sugar

2 cups gluten free flour blend

2 tablespoons sugar

½ teaspoon baking soda

1 teaspoon baking powder

½ teaspoon salt

2 tablespoons olive oil

3 eggs

1 cup coconut milk

½ cup water

1 cup shredded coconut

2 tablespoons butter

Instructions

In a small pot over medium low heat, combine berries, brown sugar and ¼ cup water. Stir and bring to a simmer. Cook for about 10 minutes or until berries begin to break down.

In a large bowl, combine flour, sugar, baking soda, baking powder and salt.

In a separate medium bowl, whisk together olive oil, eggs, coconut milk, water and shredded coconut. Add to dry ingredients and mix until just combined.

Heat a griddle or non-stick sauté pan over medium heat and add butter. Working in batches, portion batter into pan for desired size pancakes. Cook until bubbles start to form along edge. Once this happens, flip pancakes.

Serve topped with berry syrup.

Millet Breakfast Porridge

Things Needed

1 cup milk of your choice (dairy or non-dairy)

2 tablespoons honey, or to taste

2 cups cooked millet (see Chef Tips)

½ cup pineapple chunks, cut into bite sized pieces

2 tablespoons coconut flakes, toasted

½ cup pecans, chopped

Instructions

In a small saucepan, combine the milk, honey, and millet, and bring to a simmer. Continue to simmer for 3 to 5 minutes or until it reaches desired thickness.

Top with pineapple, toasted coconut, and pecans. Serve hot.

Orange Carrot Smoothie With Ginger & Dates

Things Needed

1 cup carrot, peeled and chopped

1 (2-inch) piece of fresh ginger, peeled and coarsely chopped

1 cup orange juice, preferably freshly squeezed

3 pitted dates

1 tablespoon flaxseed meal

2 ice cubes

Instructions

Combine all Things Needed in a blender. Blend until smooth. Best if served immediately.

Overnight Oatmeal With Dried Cherries

Things Needed

½ cup rolled oats

1 cup almond milk

¼ cup dried cherries

1 tablespoon chia seeds

½ teaspoon vanilla extract

½ teaspoon cinnamon

Instructions

In a container with a lid, place the oats, almond milk, cherries, chia seeds, vanilla, and cinnamon. Stir to combine and cover with the lid.

Place the container in the refrigerator overnight, at least six hours.

In the morning, remove from the refrigerator and serve cold or warm in microwave. Top with nuts or berries as desired.

Tahini & Apple Oatmeal

Things Needed

4 cups water

2 cups rolled oats

Pinch of sea salt

2 medium apples, cored, and cut into a small dice (about 2 cups)

¼ cup tahini

Instructions

Pour water into a medium pot and bring to a boil.

Once boiling, add the rolled oats, salt, and apples and turn heat down to a simmer. Cook until the oats and apples are soft, about 10 minutes. The oatmeal should be thick and the water should be absorbed.

Remove from heat. Stir in the tahini and serve immediately. (See Chef Tips.)

Vanilla Chia Pudding

Things Needed

1 cup coconut milk

1 cup Greek yogurt

2 tablespoons agave nectar

1 teaspoon vanilla extract

Dash of salt

¼ cup chia seeds

1 teaspoon lime zest

Toasted almonds for garnish (optional)

Blueberries or raspberries for garnish (optional)

Instructions

In a medium bowl, whisk together the coconut milk, Greek yogurt, agave, and vanilla until uniform.

Add salt and chia seeds and mix thoroughly.

Let the mixture sit at room temperature for 15 minutes.

Remix the pudding to reincorporate any chia seeds that settled to the bottom and add lime zest.

Cover and refrigerate for at least 3 hours.

Spoon the pudding into bowls, and garnish with almonds and fresh berries.

DELICIOUS LUNCH IDEAS FOR METABOLIC SYNDROME

Lentil Salad With Cumin & Orange Vinaigrette

Things Needed

1 teaspoon ground cumin

2 teaspoons orange zest

1 teaspoon Dijon mustard

¼ cup fresh orange juice

¼ cup olive oil

1 (16 ounce) can lentils, drained and rinsed (see Chef Tips)

½ cup carrots, shredded

½ cup celery, chopped

½ cup red pepper, chopped

¼ cup red onion, chopped

2 tablespoons parsley, chopped

Instructions

In a large bowl, whisk together cumin, orange zest, mustard, orange juice and olive oil. Season with salt and pepper.

Add lentils, carrots, celery, red pepper, red onion and parsley. Toss to combine.

Swiss Chard & Wild Rice Stuffed Squash

Things Needed

1 cup uncooked wild rice

2 cups of water

4 small acorn squash, or 2 medium size

2 tablespoons olive oil, divided

1 bunch of Swiss chard, washed and chopped

½ medium yellow onion, chopped

¾ cup chopped mushroom

½ cup chopped red pepper

¼ cup pine nuts, toasted

¼ cup of grated parmesan, divided

2 tablepoons fresh chopped parsley, divided

2 tablespoons dried currants

½ cup vegetable stock or water

Salt and pepper to taste

Instructions

Preheat oven to 400 °F. Cut acorn squash in half lengthwise, and scoop out the seeds. Brush with one tablespoon of the olive oil and sprinkle with salt and pepper. Place on a baking sheet and roast for 20 minutes, or until tender.

While squash is cooking, fill a small saucepan with 2 cups cold water, and bring to a boil. Add the wild rice. When it comes back to a boil, cover, reduce the flame to medium-low and gently simmer the rice for 30-40 minutes, or until all liquid is absorbed. Or follow package Instructions.

In a medium saucepan, pour in remaining tablespoon of olive oil. Add the peppers and onions and cook over medium heat until soft. Then add the mushrooms and Swiss chard and cook for one minute. Then add the pine nuts, stir for another minute, and take off heat.

Add cooked rice into the saucepan, along with the cheese, parsley, and currants. If mixture seems dry, add in a bit of the vegetable stock until it binds. Season with salt and pepper.

Spoon the filling into the cooked squash, and sprinkle with cheese and parsley.

Bake an additional 5 minutes until cheese is melted.

Chicken Sancocho

Things Needed

1 whole chicken, skin and solid fat removed.

4 chicken feet, toe ends clipped

12 cloves of garlic peeled and crushed, divided,

¼ cup of bitter orange juice

1½ teaspoons dried oregano

1 tablespoon salt

1 tablespoon olive oil

1 large yellow onion, diced

6 sweet ajicito peppers, cut into small dice (see Ann's Tips)

12 leaves of culantro, divided (see Ann's Tips)

10 cups of water or low sodium stock

1 cup of green plantain cut into 1-inch-dice

1 cup of yellow yautia (eddoes) cut into 1-inch-dice

1 cup yucca cut into 1-inch-dice

1 cup of carrots cut into 1-inch-long pieces

1 cup of turnip cut into 1-inch dice

4 cups kabocha cut into 1inch dice

1 cup of grated green plantain

2 tablespoons apple cider vinegar

1 tablespoon of homemade sazon

½ cup finely chopped coriander

2 sliced avocados

Instructions

Cut the chicken into 10 pieces. Set aside in a baking dish.

Make the marinade: In a small bowl, mix together 6 cloves of the garlic and the bitter orange juice. Pour over the chicken, both pieces and feet. Mix well to coat. Leave to marinate for 30 minutes. Meanwhile in a mortar, mash the remaining 6 cloves of the garlic with the oregano and salt until it forms a paste. Set aside.

Heat a large skillet over hot-medium heat. Add the chicken and the marinade. Cook until the chicken turns white and opaque. Set aside.

Heat the olive oil in a large Dutch oven over medium-low flame. Add onions, ajicitos, and half of the garlic-oregano paste. Sweat the vegetables for 7 minutes or until the onions are transparent and starting to color. Add chicken and 8 leaves of the culantro. Cook for 5 minutes. Add the water and bring to a boil. Cover. Reduce the flame to low and simmer for 15 minutes.

Add the diced plantain and cook for 10 minutes. Add the yautía, the yucca, the carrots, and the turnips. Cover and cook for 20 minutes.

Add the pumpkin and the remaining 4 culantro leaves. Cook for 15 minutes more. It should be just soft enough to mash against the side of the pan.

For the traditional presentation: Remove half of the vegetables from the sancocho with a slotted spoon and set aside. Discard the culantro leaves.

Stir the grated green plantain into the soup. Cook for 5 minutes. Return the vegetables to the pot and remove the soup from the stove. Add the apple cider vinegar and remaining garlic paste. Add the homemade 'sazon'. If necessary, add more to taste. Let the soup sit 15 minutes for the flavors to develop. Taste for salt. Ladle chicken vegetables and broth into soup plates. Serve sprinkled with the chopped cilantro, and avocado slices on the side.

Baked Falafel

Things Needed

2 tablespoons olive oil (for the baking sheet)

1 (15.5 ounce) can of chickpeas

1 red onion, cut into chunks

1-2 garlic cloves, peeled

1 cup fresh cilantro, roughly chopped

1 cup fresh parsley, roughly chopped

½ cup chickpea flour, almond flour, whole-wheat flour, or all-purpose flour

Salt and pepper, to taste

Instructions

Preheat the oven to 350 degrees. Line a baking sheet with parchment paper, then coat it with olive oil. Set aside.

Add the remaining ingredients to a blender or food processor and blend until the mixture is the consistency of a moist cookie dough. Let the mixture sit for 15 minutes.

Make 1-inch-sized balls from the mix and place on the oiled baking sheet, leaving space in between balls (should yield approximately 8 balls). Bake for 15 minutes, flipping about halfway through the cooking time. Remove the pan from the oven. Serve immediately with our Tzatziki sauce.

Brussels Sprout Pita Pizza

Things Needed

1 pound of Brussels sprouts, core removed and thinly sliced

¼ cup minced red onion

2 tablespoons olive oil, divided

1 can of cannellini beans, drained and rinsed

¼ cup tahini

½ teaspoon cumin

1 lemon, zested and juiced

4 whole wheat pitas

Salt and pepper to taste

Instructions

Preheat oven to 400°F. Line a baking sheet with parchment paper.

In a bowl, mix the shredded Brussel sprouts and red onion with 1 tablespoon of the olive oil. When the vegetables are lightly coated with oil, tip onto the prepared baking sheet, and spread out into a single, even layer. Do not crowd. Season with salt and pepper.

Roast for about 10 minutes, or until the Brussel sprouts are soft and lightly browned.

Meanwhile in bowl of a food processor, puree cannellini beans, tahini, cumin, lemon juice, and zest. Season with salt and pepper to taste.

Place pita on a baking sheet and warm slightly in oven. Remove and spread a portion of the bean spread onto each pita and top with a portion of the shredded Brussel sprouts. Drizzle with any remaining olive oil.

Cut each pita into four slices and serve.

Eggplant Pita Pizza

Things Needed

1 large eggplant, medium diced

2 tablespoons olive oil

1 can of cannellini beans, drained and rinsed

¼ cup tahini

½ teaspoon cumin

1 lemon, juiced and zested

4 whole wheat pitas

Salt and pepper to taste

¼ teaspoon red pepper flakes

Parsley or cilantro for garnish, chopped

Instructions

Preheat oven to 400°F.

On a baking sheet, place the eggplant in a single layer. Drizzle the eggplant with olive oil and season with salt and pepper.

Place the eggplant in the oven and bake for about 20 minutes, or until the eggplant is soft and golden brown.

In the bowl of a food processor, place the cannellini beans, tahini, cumin, lemon juice, and zest. Puree the beans until smooth. Season with salt and pepper to taste.

Place the pita on a baking sheet and warm slightly in the oven. Remove from the oven and spread a portion of the bean spread onto each pita. Top with roasted eggplant and sprinkled with red pepper flakes and garnished with chopped parsley or cilantro.

Cut each pita into four slices and serve

Sweet Potato Chickpea Bowl

Things Needed

1 small red onion, quartered

2 large sweet potatoes, halved

3 tablespoons olive oil, divided

1 (15-ounce) can chickpeas, drained, rinsed and patted dry

1 teaspoon cumin

¾ teaspoon chili powder

¾ teaspoon garlic powder

½ teaspoon oregano

¼ teaspoon turmeric

salt and pepper to taste

¼ cup tahini

1 tablespoon maple syrup

½ lemon, juiced

2-4 tablespoons hot water, as needed

1 cup raw spinach leaves, packed

2 cups cooked farro

Instructions

Preheat the oven to 400 °F.

Coat the red onion and sweet potatoes with 2 tablespoons olive oil. Sprinkle with salt and pepper. Roast the vegetables in the oven for about 20 minutes, or until fork tender. Then, remove them from oven and cool to room temperature.

While the vegetables are roasting, toss the chickpeas, cumin, chili powder, garlic powder, oregano, turmeric and salt and pepper in a medium-sized bowl.

Heat a medium-sized skillet over medium-high heat. Add the oil and the chickpea mixture. Cook the chickpeas until they are brown and fragrant, stirring frequently, about 8-10 minutes. Set aside. (See Chef Tips)

To make the tahini sauce, stir together the tahini, maple syrup and lemon juice. If the mixture is too thick to pour easily (molasses like), add a tablespoon of water and stir. Repeat this process until you have a pourable mixture.

Once the three components are finished, the roasted vegetables, chickpeas and tahini, put the spinach in a layer at the bottom of a medium sized bowl. Then put the farro (or rice) on top. Follow this with the vegetables and chickpeas. Pour the tahini sauce on top.

Vegetarian Shepherd's Pie

Things Needed

2 pounds Yukon gold or Idaho potatoes, cut into quarters

3 tablespoons butter

¾ cups uncooked brown or green lentils, rinsed

2 cups vegetable stock

1 teaspoon fresh thyme leaves

1 teaspoon fresh rosemary leaves

½ cup diced celery

½ cup diced carrots

½ cup sliced green beans

½ cup corn kernels

Salt and pepper to taste

Instructions

Preheat oven to 400°F.

In a large sauce pot, place the potatoes and cover with water. Bring pot to a soft boil and cover. Let cook for 20-30 minutes, or until potatoes are soft when poked with a knife or fork.

Drain the potatoes, reserving about 1 cup of the water. Mash the potatoes with a fork or pastry cutter, then add butter. Add the reserved water to achieve desired texture for mashed potatoes. Season with salt and pepper and set aside.

While the potatoes are boiling, place the lentils, vegetable stock, thyme, and rosemary in another sauce pot. Bring to a boil, then reduce the heat to simmer. Cook the lentils until tender and almost all the stock has been absorbed, about 30-40 minutes.

Add the celery, carrots, green beans, and corn to the lentils and cook all together for about 10 minutes, or until the vegetables are soft. Season with salt and pepper.

In a lightly greased 9x9 inch baking dish, scoop in the lentil and vegetable mixture. Add the mashed potatoes on top and flatten.

Place in the oven for about 10 minutes, or until the mashed potatoes become lightly golden brown.

Curried Chickpea Patties

Things Needed

1 (15.5 ounce) can chickpeas, drained and rinsed

1 small onion, about ½ cup, chopped

1 clove of garlic, minced

4 eggs

½ cup breadcrumbs

¼ cup flat-leaf parsley, chopped

2 teaspoons lemon zest

½ teaspoon paprika

2 teaspoons curry powder

2 tablespoons olive oil

Whole-wheat pita pockets or large lettuce leaves (optional, for serving)

For the yogurt sauce:

½ cup Greek yogurt

1 teaspoon lemon zest

1 tablespoon lemon juice

1 teaspoon fresh mint, chopped

Salt and pepper, to taste

Instructions

Combine chickpeas, onions, garlic, and eggs in a food processor. Blend until the mixture has the texture of a chunky hummus, leaving some large chickpea pieces.

Transfer the chickpea mixture to a large bowl and combine with the remaining ingredients. Mix well. Form into 4 patties or up to 12 small patties if you want to eat in a pita pocket or lettuce wrap. The mixture should be very wet to ensure a moist patty, but if you are having trouble forming them, stir in more breadcrumbs, 1 tablespoon at a time.

Combine all Things Needed for the yogurt sauce. Taste for seasoning and set aside.

Heat 2 tablespoons of olive oil in a skillet over medium heat. Drop the patties into the pan with space in between. Do this in batches if necessary. Cook for 5 minutes, then carefully flip and cook the other side for another 5 minutes or until golden and cooked through. Serve on a warm pita pocket or in a lettuce wrap with the yogurt sauce.

Granola-Stuffed Winter Squash

Things Needed

2 small acorn squash or 1 butternut squash

2 tablespoons olive oil or melted butter

1 tablespoon of brown sugar

1 ½ cups of granola and/or oats (see Chef Tips)

3 tablespoons of raisins

½ cup walnuts, chopped + 1 tablespoon for garnish

½ cup hot water

½ cup maple syrup, or to taste, divided

Instructions

Preheat the oven to 425 degrees. Cut the squash in half lengthwise, and scoop out the seeds and reserve in a bowl for later use.

Using a brush, spread the olive oil or melted butter all over the cut sides of the squash, then sprinkle with brown sugar. Place cut side up on a baking sheet lined with aluminum foil. Bake for 20-25 minutes or until nearly tender.

While the squash halves bake, make the stuffing: In a large bowl mix together the granola, oats, raisins, and the ½ cup of chopped walnuts. Add ½ cup of hot water and ¼ cup of the maple syrup. Mix well. Set aside, and clean the seeds so that minimal meat or strings are attached.

When the squash halves are soft, take them out of the oven and stuff the insides with the granola mixture. With a brush, slather some of the remaining maple syrup on top. Put them back on the baking sheet along with the reserved squash seeds.

Return to the oven and bake at 425 degrees oven for another 10 minutes, or until the squash halves are completely tender when pierced with a fork or skewer. Serve warm, garnished with walnuts and the toasted acorn squash seeds.

Kale & Lemon Barlotto

Things Needed

3 tablespoons olive oil

6 medium shallots or ½ onion, minced

3 garlic cloves, minced

Salt and pepper, to taste

2 cups pearled barley

7 cups of hot stock

2 tablespoons lemon juice

2 lemons, zested

½ cup Parmesan cheese, plus more for garnish

½ cup plain Greek yogurt

4 cups kale leaves, chopped

¼ cup walnuts, chopped toasted

Instructions

Heat the olive oil in a large, heavy saucepan over medium heat. Add the shallots or onions, garlic and salt and sauté, stirring constantly for about 4 minutes or until the onions begin to soften. Do not let brown.

Add the barley to the pot and stir well. Add 1 cup of stock and 2 tablespoons of lemon juice and simmer for 3 to 4 minutes, until the barley has almost absorbed all the liquid.

1 cup at a time, add the remaining 6 cups of stock, letting the barley absorb most of the stock before adding in more. Stir often, it should take about 30 minutes. Taste the barley to test for doneness.

Once the barley is tender, stir in the lemon zest, Parmesan cheese, yogurt and kale leaves. Continue to cook stirring until the kale is a bright green. Taste for seasoning, then serve with chopped walnuts and some extra grated Parmesan.

Moroccan Vegetable Stew

Things Needed

4 cups vegetable broth or water

1 teaspoon sea salt, or to taste

3 cloves garlic, smashed and peeled

1 bay leaf

1 small cinnamon stick (see Chef Tips)

1 inch ginger root, split in half lengthwise (see Chef Tips)

½ teaspoon saffron threads dissolved in a tablespoon of boiling water

1 inch strip of lemon peel (optional)

1 whole dried chipotle pepper (optional)

3 to 4 small turnips, peeled and quartered

3 to 4 medium carrots, scrubbed and cut into
½-inch chunks

2 small kohlrabi bulbs, peeled and quartered
(see Chef Tips)

5 small Yukon Gold potatoes, quartered

1 (14 ounce) can diced tomatoes

1 red bell pepper, deseeded and cut into 1-inch
chunks

4 sticks celery, quartered

2 cups kabocha or butternut squash, cut into 1-
inch cubes

1 (14 ounce) can chickpeas, drained and rinsed
(see Chef Tips)

½ cup frozen lima beans

½ cup flat leaf parsley, chopped

½ cup cilantro or mint, chopped

Harissa (optional)

Instructions

Bring the broth or water to a boil in a large pot. Add the salt, garlic, bay leaf, cinnamon stick, ginger, saffron threads, lemon peel and chipotle pepper, if using. Use a tablespoon of broth to rinse the saffron bowl so that you get every last thread. Cook for 2 minutes.

Add the turnips, carrots, kohlrabi, potatoes, and diced tomatoes to the broth. Mix well. Bring back to a boil, cover, then turn the heat down to medium-low and simmer for 30 minutes.

Add the bell pepper, celery, and squash. Mix in. Cook covered until the squash is just tender, about 15 to 20 minutes.

Add the chickpeas and lima beans. Cook until heated through. Taste for salt. Stir in the chopped herbs, cover, and cook 1 minute more. Turn off the heat and let the stew steam for 5 to 10 minutes. Remove and discard the bay leaf, ginger, chipotle pepper and cinnamon stick before serving. Serve with couscous or quinoa.

Refried Beans, Pico and Sunny Side Egg Breakfast Toast

Things Needed

1 slice whole grain bread

2 Tbsp. refried beans, low sodium

1 Tbsp. pico de gallo

1 sunny side up egg

Instructions

Toast bread.

Warm beans on stovetop or in a microwave.

Cook egg sunny-side up.

Top all ingredients onto toast.

Citrus Quinoa Avocado Salad

Things Needed

For the salad:

½ cup cucumber, diced

1 cup cherry tomatoes, cut in half

2 small cloves garlic, minced

¼ cup red onion, chopped

1 bunch cilantro

2 cups spinach, thinly sliced

1 (15.5 ounce) can garbanzo beans, no-salt-added or low-sodium (drained and rinsed)

1 cup cooked and cooled quinoa

2 medium avocados, diced

For the dressing:

Juice of 2 lemons

Zest of 1 lemon

2 teaspoon Dijon mustard

1 tablespoon olive oil

1 teaspoon honey

½ teaspoon ground cumin

Dash of cayenne pepper (optional)

Salt and pepper, to taste

Instructions

Place all salad Things Needed in a bowl.

Whisk all dressing Things Needed together in a separate bowl.

Drizzle dressing over salad mixture and gently toss ingredients together until dressing is incorporated throughout.

Cocoa Cherry Protein Shake

Things Needed

¾ cup whole milk

¼ cup Greek yogurt

½ cup frozen cherries

1 tbsp protein powder (see Chef Notes)

1 tbsp unsweetened cocoa powder

1 tbsp nut butter

1 tbsp flaxseed meal

½ cup ice

Instructions

Add all Things Needed to a high-speed blender and blend on high until smooth.

Serve immediately.

Avocado & Egg Toast

Things Needed

1/2 avocado, ripe

2 slices whole grain toast

Salt and pepper, to taste

Cayenne, to taste (optional)

Squeeze of lime (optional)

1 hard-boiled egg, sliced

Instructions

Scoop out the avocado flesh and spread it onto the toast by mashing it with the back of a fork.

Sprinkle salt, pepper, cayenne and squeeze of lime. Then layer hard-boiled egg slices on top of the avocado mash, and sprinkle with a little more salt and pepper.

Easy Quinoa Porridge With Golden Milk

Things Needed

1⅓ cups cooked quinoa (see Chef Tips)

1 cups 2% milk, or nondairy milk of choice

Pinch of sea salt

2 tablespoons cranberries

3 dates, pitted and chopped

1 teaspoon ginger root, freshly grated

½ teaspoon turmeric root, freshly grated (see Chef Tips)

1 cup apple, grated

⅓ cup fresh blueberries (optional)

2 tablespoons almonds, dry toasted and sliced

Plain Greek yogurt for serving (optional)

Instructions

In a small pot over medium-high heat, add the quinoa, milk, and a pinch of sea salt. Stir to mix. Add the cranberries, dates, grated ginger root, and turmeric. Stir again. Bring to a boil, cover, and turn the heat down to low. Cook for 5 to 8 minutes, stirring from time to time. For a thicker porridge, crack the lid.

Stir in the grated apple. Mix well. Cover and cook 2 to 3 minutes more. Add the blueberries and stir to mix. Cover, turn off the heat, and let sit for 2 to 3 minutes while you toast the nuts.

To dry toast the nuts: Heat a small heavy frying pan over medium-high heat. Add the nuts and cook, shaking until they are a light golden color — about 2 to 3 minutes. As soon as they are pale gold, turn off the heat, as there will be enough heat left to finish the toasting.

Serve the porridge in bowls with sprinkled with nuts and either with a dollop of plain Greek yogurt, if using, or with extra cold milk poured over it.

Chickpea Salad Sandwich

Things Needed

for 3 servings

15 oz chickpeas (425 g), 1 can, drained and rinsed

¼ cup red onion (40 g), diced

½ red bell pepper, diced

3 tablespoons vegan mayonnaise

½ teaspoon dijon mustard

½ teaspoon garlic powder

½ teaspoon onion powder

salt, to taste

pepper, to taste

1 tablespoon fresh dill, chopped

leafy green, to serve

bread, sliced, to serve

Instructions

In a medium mixing bowl, add chickpeas and mash with potato masher until a chunky texture is reached.

Add the red onion, red pepper, vegan mayo, Dijon mustard, garlic powder, onion powder, salt, pepper, and dill, and stir until well combined.

Store chickpea salad in refrigerator for up to five days. To assemble sandwich, spread mixture onto bread and top with leafy greens of choice.

Wrap in parchment paper and secure with rubber band.

Enjoy!

Honey Mustard Chicken Salad

Things Needed

for 4 servings

⅓ cup honey (115 g)

¼ cup dijon mustard (65 g)

2 tablespoons olive oil

2 cloves garlic, minced

2 teaspoons salt

1 teaspoon pepper

4 boneless, skinless chicken thighs

¼ cup bacon (60 g), chopped

4 cups romaine lettuce (300 g), chopped

1 cup cherry tomatoes (200 g), halved

¼ red onion, sliced

1 avocado, pitted and sliced

Instructions

In a small bowl or liquid measuring cup, mix the honey, mustard, oil, garlic, salt, and pepper.

Place the chicken thighs in a dish and pour the marinade over the chicken, reserving half for later.

Flip the chicken thighs over, fully covering them in the marinade.

Cover the dish with plastic wrap and refrigerate for 30 minutes to an hour.

Heat a large skillet over medium heat, and place the chicken thighs in the pan.

Cook for five minutes on each side, or until the chicken is cooked through.

Remove the chicken and set aside.

Wipe the pan clean and place back on the heat.

Add the chopped bacon to the pan and cook until crispy, about ten minutes.

Transfer the bacon to a paper towel-lined plate to drain.

Add three tablespoons of water to the reserved marinade and stir to combine.

Slice the chicken into strips.

Add the romaine, cherry tomatoes, red onion, avocado, cooked bacon, and chicken to a bowl and drizzle with the remaining honey mustard dressing.

Enjoy!

Chicken Enchilada-Stuffed Zucchini Boats

Things Needed

for 1 serving

1 boneless, skinless chicken breast, sliced into ½-inch (1 cm) pieces

½ teaspoon salt

¼ teaspoon ground black pepper

½ teaspoon chili powder

2 teaspoons olive oil

½ cup salsa (130 g), mild

1 zucchini, cut in half lengthwise, centers hollowed out

2 tablespoons shredded cheddar cheese

1 roma tomato, diced

¼ avocado, dinced

2 tablespoons chopped cilantro

1 lime, cut into wedges

Lime Crema

½ cup nonfat greek yogurt (140 g), plain

1 tablespoon lime juice

¼ teaspoon salt

Instructions

Preheat oven to 375°F (190°C).

Cut zucchini in half and hollow out the centers

Add the Greek yogurt, lime juice, and salt together in a small bowl and stir to combine.

On a cutting board, season the chicken breast with salt, pepper, and chili powder.

Heat olive oil in a large pan over medium heat. Once the oil begins to shimmer, add the chicken and cook until browned, about 3 minutes.

Remove the chicken from the pan and let cool. Once cooled, shred the chicken with a fork.

Add the chicken to a bowl with the salsa and stir to combine.

Stuff chicken mixture in hollowed out zucchini boats, and top with cheddar cheese.

Bake until cheese is melted and browned, and zucchini is tender, about 20 minutes.

Top with tomato, avocado, cilantro, and lime crema. Serve with lime wedges.

Enjoy!

Ham & Cheese Chicken Rollups

Things Needed

for 4 servings

2 boneless, skinless chicken breasts

1 teaspoon salt, for chicken

¼ teaspoon pepper, for chicken

1 teaspoon garlic powder

4 slices ham

4 slices provolone cheese

1 cup flour (125 g)

2 eggs, beaten

1 cup breadcrumb (115 g)

3 cups broccoli floret (450 g)

4 tablespoons olive oil

1 teaspoon salt

¼ teaspoon pepper

Instructions

Preheat oven to 400°F (200°C)

Cut about ¾ of the way through the chicken horizontally, making sure not to cut through the other side. Flip the chicken open and flat.

Lay a sheet of plastic wrap on top of the chicken and pound it flatter using a pot or a pan. Remove the plastic wrap.

Season with the salt, pepper, and garlic powder, rubbing the seasoning in evenly. Lay 2-3 slices of ham over the chicken, followed by 4 slices of provolone cheese.

Carefully roll the chicken up.

Transfer the flour, eggs, and breadcrumbs into 3 separate bowls.

Dip the chicken roll into the flour, tapping off any excess, and then into the egg, followed by the breadcrumbs. Place on a baking sheet

Add the broccoli to the baking sheet, mixing it with the olive oil, salt, and pepper. Make sure to save a little oil to drizzle on top of the chicken.

Bake for 20 minutes.

Slice, then serve!

Enjoy!

Portobello Fajita Bowl Meal Prep

Things Needed

for 4 servings

1 yellow bell pepper

1 red bell pepper

1 green bell pepper

1 teaspoon salt, divided

½ teaspoon cumin, divided

1 teaspoon smoked paprika, divided

1 ½ teaspoons chili powder, divided

1 teaspoon red pepper flakes, divided

4 portobello mushrooms

1 tablespoon oil

1 large white onion

3 cloves garlic, minced

3 cups brown rice (675 g), cooked

1 cup pico de gallo (240 g)

1 cup black beans (60 g), drained and rinsed

1 cup corn (165 g)

1 cup shredded cheddar cheese (100 g)

1 avocado, sliced

1 lime, sliced into wedges

fresh cilantro, for garnish

Instructions

Slice the stem off of the peppers so that they will stand steadily when flipped upside down. Slice the peppers into quarters from the bottom to the top around the core and seeds. Slice each quarter into 1-inch (2 ½ cm) thick slices. Transfer to a large bowl.

Add ½ teaspoon salt, ¼ teaspoon cumin, ½ teaspoon smoked paprika, 1 teaspoon chili powder, and ½ teaspoon red pepper flakes. Toss to coat the peppers evenly in the spices and set aside.

Remove the stems from the portobello mushrooms and slice into 1-inch-wide (2 cm) pieces, then transfer a large bowl.

Add the remaining ½ teaspoon salt, ½ teaspoon chili powder, ½ teaspoon smoked paprika, ¼ teaspoon cumin, and ½ teaspoon red pepper flakes. Toss to coat the mushrooms evenly in the spices and set aside.

Thinly slice the onion.

Heat oil in a large cast-iron pan over medium-high heat. Add the onion and cook, stirring occasionally, until translucent, about 3 minutes. Add the garlic and bell peppers, and cook for about 5 more minutes, stirring constantly until peppers are tender. Remove the pepper and onion mixture from the pan and set aside.

Add the mushrooms to the skillet and cook until the mushrooms are tender, stirring constantly, about 5 minutes

Divide the brown rice between 4 food storage containers. Top each container with pico de gallo, black beans, corn, cheddar cheese, the cooked bell peppers and onions, and the sliced portobello. Garnish with an avocado slice, a lime wedge, and cilantro.

Store in the refrigerator for up to 4 days.

Enjoy!

Tofu Stir Fry

Things Needed

for 2 servings

4 cloves garlic, minced, divided

2 teaspoons fresh ginger, grated

1 tablespoon honey

1 teaspoon sriracha

¼ cup lime juice (60 mL)

¼ cup reduced sodium soy sauce (60 mL)

1 block extra firm tofu

2 tablespoons sesame oil

1 cup sliced white onion

1 cup sliced carrot

1 cup sliced red bell pepper

½ cup edamame (75 g), frozen, thawed

3 cups soba noodle (300 g), cooked

1 tablespoon sesame seed

green onion, chopped, to serve

Instructions

In a medium bowl, mix together 2 cloves of garlic, the ginger, honey, Sriracha, lime juice, and soy sauce. Set aside.

Wrap the tofu in a dish towel, then place a plate on top. Let drain for 10-15 minutes, then remove the plate, unwrap the tofu, and slice into cubes.

In a wok or large frying pan, heat the sesame oil over medium heat. Add the tofu and pan fry for 5-7 minutes, stirring occasionally.

Add the remaining 2 cloves of minced garlic and the onion and stir until softened, about 1 minute.

Add the carrot, bell pepper, and edamame and cook, stirring occasionally, until tender, 2-3 minutes.

Add the soba noodles, reserved sauce, and sesame seeds. Cook for 1-2 minutes, stirring occasionally, until warmed through. Remove the pan from the heat.

Garnish with green onions, if desired.

Enjoy!

Sheet Tray Fajitas Rice Bowl

Things Needed

for 1 serving

¼ cup brown rice (50 g)

1 teaspoon salt, divided

¾ cup water (180 mL)

4 oz flank steak (115 g), thinly sliced

1 small red onion, thinly sliced

1 red bell pepper, thinly sliced lengthwise

1 tablespoon lime juice

1 teaspoon onion powder

¾ teaspoon chili powder

½ teaspoon ground black pepper

2 tablespoons fresh cilantro, chopped

1 lime, cut into wedges

Instructions

Preheat oven to 450°F (230°C).

Place the rice in a sieve and rinse under cold water to remove excess starch.

Transfer the rice to a small pot with salt and water and bring to a boil over high heat. Reduce to a simmer, put a lid on, and cook until water is absorbed, about 45 minutes.

In a bowl, add the skirt steak, red onion, bell pepper, lime juice, onion powder, chili powder, black pepper, and remaining salt and toss until well combined.

Transfer to a parchment paper-lined sheet tray and bake for 12 to 15 minutes.

Serve steak over rice and top with cilantro and lime wedges.

Enjoy!

Eggplant Parmesan Boats

Things Needed

for 4 servings

2 medium eggplants

2 tablespoons olive oil

salt, to taste

pepper, to taste

½ lb ground turkey (225 g)

1 onion, diced

2 cups marinara sauce (520 g)

2 cloves garlic, minced

1 cup shredded low-fat mozzarella (100 g)

½ cup grated parmesan cheese (55 g)

fresh basil, for garnish

Instructions

Preheat oven to 400°F (200°C).

Scoop out inside of eggplant leaving about ½-inch (1 cm) border inside.

Chop the remaining eggplant and reserve.

Brush the scooped out eggplants with olive oil, sprinkle with salt and pepper.

Bake for 10-15 minutes.

Heat olive oil in medium skillet over medium heat.

Add onions and garlic to the pan. Cook until translucent. Add ground turkey and season with garlic powder, salt and pepper. Cook until the meat is browned.

Add leftover eggplant pieces to ground turkey and onion. Cook for 5-8 minutes or until tender.

Add marinara sauce and cook for another 3-5 minutes.

Scoop meat sauce into the eggplants and sprinkle with mozzarella and parmesan.

Bake for 10-15 minutes, or until cheese is melted.

Sprinkle with basil and serve.

Enjoy!

Lentil & Roasted Vegetable Salad

Things Needed

for 2 servings

2 cups butternut squash (410 g), cubed

2 cups brussels sprouts (200 g), quartered

1 red onion, cut into wedges

1 tablespoon olive oil

salt, to taste

pepper, to taste

1 cup green lentil (170 g), rinsed

3 cups water (720 mL), or vegetable broth

3 tablespoons balsamic vinegar

1 tablespoon maple syrup

salt, to taste

pepper, to taste

Instructions

Preheat oven to 400°F (200°C).

Add butternut squash, Brussels sprouts, and red onion to to a parchment paper-lined baking sheet. Season with olive oil, salt, and pepper, and use hands to mix until seasoning is fully distributed.

Bake for 20 minutes, flipping halfway through.

In a medium saucepan, add lentils and water, and bring to a boil.

Reduce heat to a simmer and cover for 20-25 minutes or until lentils are tender. Drain excess water if necessary.

When vegetables are finished roasting, transfer to a mixing bowl and add lentils.

For the dressing, combine balsamic vinegar, maple syrup, salt, and pepper in liquid measuring cup and whisk until combined.

Pour dressing over lentils and vegetables and toss until fully coated.

Transfer lentil salad to two containers and refrigerate for up to 5 days.

Enjoy!

Zucchini "Enchiladas"

Things Needed

for 5 servings

2 tablespoons olive oil

½ yellow onion, diced

2 cloves garlic, minced

1 can black beans, drained and rinsed

1 can corn, drained and rinsed

1 ½ cups enchilada sauce (435 g), divided

½ lime, juiced

1 teaspoon salt

1 teaspoon cumin

½ teaspoon chili powder

4 zucchinis

½ cup shredded cheddar cheese (50 g)

sour cream, for serving

fresh cilantro, for serving

Instructions

Preheat oven to 375°F (190°C).

In a pan over medium heat, add the oil and the onions and cook until the onions are translucent.

Add the garlic and stir to combine.

Add the black beans, corn, 1 cup (290 g) of enchilada sauce, lime juice, salt, cumin, and chili powder, and stir until combined. Cook until just simmering. Set aside.

Cut off the end of each zucchini then using a vegetable peeler, peel each zucchini into wide strips.

Place 4-5 zucchini strips on a plate and spoon a large spoonful of filling at the bottom of the strips.

Fold the ends of the zucchini over the filling and continue to roll, tightly.

Transfer the zucchini rolls to a baking dish.

Spoon over the remaining enchilada sauce and top with cheese.

Bake for 15-20 minutes or until cheese is melted.

Serve with sour cream and cilantro.

Enjoy!

Cauliflower Walnut Burritos

Things Needed

for 4 servings

½ head cauliflower, broken into florets

¾ cup walnuts (75 g)

olive oil, to taste

½ medium yellow onion, diced

2 cloves garlic, minced

2 ½ teaspoons chili powder

1 teaspoon ground cumin

½ teaspoon smoked paprika

2 tablespoons low sodium soy sauce

¼ cup low sodium vegetable broth (60 mL)

kosher salt, to taste

pepper, to taste

4 large flour tortillas

2 cups spanish rice (460 g), cooked

lettuce, chopped, for serving

tomato, diced, for serving

shredded vegan cheddar cheese, for serving

guacamole, for serving

Instructions

Add the cauliflower florets and walnuts to a food processor and pulse until crumbly. Set aside.

Heat a drizzle of olive oil in a large saucepan over medium heat. Once the oil begins to shimmer, add the onion and cook for 3-4 minutes, until semi-translucent. Add the cauliflower mixture and cook for 4-5 minutes, until the cauliflower is semi-tender.

Add another drizzle of olive oil, the garlic, chili powder, cumin, paprika, and soy sauce and cook for 2-3 minutes more, until the spices are fragrant. Add the vegetable broth and cook for another 5-6 minutes, until the broth has evaporated and the cauliflower is tender. Season with salt and pepper to taste.

To assemble a burrito, add ¼ of the Spanish rice, ¼ of the cauliflower-walnut mixture, some lettuce, tomatoes, vegan cheese, and guacamole to the center of a tortilla. Fold in the sides and roll up, keeping the filling tucked in place. Repeat with the remaining Things Needed. Cut in half and serve.

Enjoy!

Healthier Veggie Fried Rice

Things Needed

for 2 servings

2 cups brown rice (390 g)

2 cups vegetable broth (475 mL)

2 carrots, diced

1 tablespoon oil

½ white onion, diced

2 cloves garlic, minced

½ cup frozen peas (75 g)

salt, to taste

pepper, to taste

2 eggs, whisked

scallion, sliced, for garnish

Instructions

Add the brown rice, vegetable broth, and diced carrots to your Instant Pot. Stir until combined.

Close the lid until you hear the beep. Tip: Closing the lid can be tricky. Have the pressure knob at 11 o'clock and turn right.

Turn pressure knob to "Sealing". Select Manual and reduce the time to 24 minutes. It will say "On" in a few seconds. Note: the Instant Pot will need to warm up for 5-10 minutes. Steam will be released and a few minutes later, the time will start counting down.

Once the time goes off, carefully turn the pressure knob to "Venting". Let all of the stream release before opening the lid.

Stir the rice, then transfer from the pot into a medium sized bowl and set aside.

Select "Saute" on the Instant Pot. Once it says "Hot", add the oil.

When the oil is shimmering, add the onion. Cook for around 1 minute until slightly opaque.

Add the minced garlic, frozen peas, salt, and pepper. Mix until incorporated.

Add rice mixture and stir until everything is combined.

Make a well in the middle of the rice for the eggs. Pour the beaten eggs into the well, stirring only the eggs until they are cooked.

Mix everything together. Top with scallions.

Enjoy!

TASTY DINNERTIME DISHES FOR METABOLIC SYNDROME

Vegan Lasagna Soup

Things Needed

for 6 servings

1 tablespoon olive oil

1 onion, diced

3 cloves garlic, minced

2 tablespoons tomato paste

1 teaspoon dried basil

1 teaspoon dried oregano

28 oz crushed tomato (795 g)

6 cups vegetable broth (1.4 L)

⅓ cup green lentil (50 g), rinsed

8 oz lasagna noodle (225 g), uncooked

3 cups spinach (120 g)

fresh basil, cut chiffonade, for serving

Instructions

In a large pot, heat the olive oil over medium heat. Once the oil begins to shimmer, add the onion and cook for 3-4 minutes, until semi-translucent.

Add the garlic, tomato paste, basil, and oregano, and cook for 2-3 more minutes, or until the onions are translucent and herbs are fragrant.

Add the crushed tomatoes, vegetable broth, and lentils, and bring to a boil. Increase heat to medium-high and cook for 10 minutes or until lentils are halfway tender.

Break apart the lasagna noodles into about 2-inch-long (5-cm) pieces and add to the pot. Let the soup cook for another 10-15 minutes, or until the pasta is al dente and the lentils are tender.

Stir in the spinach and let wilt, then serve immediately.

Enjoy!

Whole Wheat Pasta With Lemon Kale Chicken

Things Needed

for 2 servings

4 oz whole wheat spaghetti (115 g)

1 boneless, skinless chicken breast, cubed

5 tablespoons extra virgin olive oil

2 cloves garlic, minced

¼ teaspoon red pepper flakes

2 cups curly kale (135 g), chopped, ribs removed

1 lemon lemon zest

1 tablespoon lemon juice

kosher salt, to taste

ground black pepper, to taste

Instructions

Boil salted water and cook the pasta for 1 minute less than the time indicated on the package. When the pasta is finished cooking, reserve ¼ cup (60 ml) of pasta water.

Meanwhile, heat two tablespoons of olive oil in a cast-iron skillet. Season cubed chicken with salt and pepper, add it to the skillet, and brown it on each side. Once cooked through — about 2 to 4 minutes — remove from skillet and reserve.

Heat remaining three tablespoons of olive oil in skillet and add garlic and red pepper flakes. Cook until fragrant, about 1 minutes.

Add kale, lemon zest, lemon juice, salt, and reserved pasta water. Cook until kale is tender, about 3 minutes.

Add cooked chicken, and pasta. Stir to coat, and serve immediately.

Enjoy!

Fajita Pasta Bake

Things Needed

for 6 servings

1 yellow bell pepper, seeded and sliced

1 green bell pepper, seeded and sliced

1 red bell pepper, seeded and sliced

2 ½ cups mushroom (185 g), sliced

1 medium yellow onion, diced

1 tablespoon chili powder

1 tablespoon paprika

1 tablespoon garlic powder

1 tablespoon cumin

1 teaspoon salt

1 teaspoon pepper

3 tablespoons olive oil

4 cups penne pasta (400 g), uncooked

1 ½ cups sour cream (345 g)

3 cups shredded pepper jack cheese (300 g)

fresh parsley, chopped. for garnish

Instructions

Preheat the oven to 400°F (200°C).

In a nonstick baking dish, add the bell peppers, mushrooms, and onion.

In a small bowl, combine the chili powder, paprika, garlic powder, cumin, salt, and pepper.

Pour the olive oil and half of the spice mix over the vegetables and toss well to coat.

Bake the vegetables for about 30 minutes, stirring occasionally, until tender.

In a large pot of boiling water, cook the pasta according to the package instructions, until tender.

Drain the pasta, reserving about 1 cup (240 ml) of cooking water.

Return the drained pasta to the pot and add the roasted vegetables. Add the rest of the spice mix, the reserved pasta water, and the sour cream and mix to combine.

Transfer the pasta mixture to the baking dish used for roasting the vegetables and spread evenly. Sprinkle the cheese over the top.

Bake for about 15 minutes, until the cheese is golden brown.

Let cool for about 5 minutes, then serve. Garnish with parsley, if desired.

Enjoy!

Loaded Baked Potato Soup

Things Needed

for 6 servings

4 lb russet potato (1.8 g), washed

1 tablespoon olive oil

1 teaspoon salt

½ teaspoon pepper

1 onion, diced

3 cloves garlic

3 tablespoons butter

¼ cup flour (30 g)

2 ½ cups chicken broth (590 mL)

8 oz cream cheese (225 g)

Garnish

shredded cheese

bacon, diced

fresh chive, chopped

Instructions

Preheat your oven to 425°F (220°C).

On a parchment paper-lined baking sheet, rub potatoes with salt, pepper, and olive oil.

Bake in preheated oven for 40-50 minutes.

Once cooled, peel and mash potatoes, and set aside.

Heat oil in large pot over a medium-high heat.

Add onion and garlic. Cook until translucent and garlic is fragant, about 5 minutes.

Add butter and melt.

Bring in flour and stir until mixture is lightly browned.

Add in the chicken broth and cream cheese. Stir until fully incorporated

Add in the mashed potatoes and combine.

Season with salt and pepper.

Garnish bowl with shredded cheese, bacon, and chives.

Enjoy!

Penne Alla Vodka Pasta

Things Needed

for 3 servings

2 tablespoons olive oil

1 onion, chopped

1 lb ground beef (455 g)

1 teaspoon salt

1 teaspoon pepper

28 oz crushed tomato (795 g), 1 can

½ cup vodka (120 mL)

½ teaspoon red chili flake

½ cup heavy cream (120 mL)

4 cups penne pasta (400 g)

fresh parsley, to garnish

½ cup Parmesan (110 g), to garnish

Instructions

Heat oil in a large pot over high heat. Cook onion until translucent.

Add beef, salt, and pepper, cooking until all the moisture has evaporated and the beef is browned.

Add crushed tomatoes, vodka, and chili flakes, stirring and cooking until half of the liquid has evaporated and the sauce has reduced.

Add cream, stirring until evenly incorporated.

Stir in pasta until evenly coated.

Serve with parsley and parmesan.

Nutrition Calories: 1753 Fat: 69 grams Carbs: 193 grams Fiber: 13 grams Sugars: 22 grams Protein: 93 grams

Enjoy!

Chorizo Tomato Rotini Pasta

Things Needed

for 3 servings

1 tablespoon oil

4 oz chorizo (110 g), chopped

½ onion, chopped

1 lb ground beef (455 g)

2 teaspoons salt

2 teaspoons pepper

3 cups tomato sauce (450 g)

1 ¼ cups rotini pasta (250 g)

½ cup parmesan cheese (50 g)

½ cup fresh basil (12 g), chopped

Instructions

Heat oil in a large pot over medium-high heat.

Cook chorizo until slightly crispy.

Add the onions and cook until translucent.

Add the beef, salt, and pepper, cooking until no pink is showing.

Pour in the tomato sauce, and cook until sauce thickens.

Add the pasta, parmesan, and basil, stirring until the pasta is evenly coated.

Enjoy!

Spinach Mushroom Pesto Spaghetti

Things Needed

for 2 servings

1 tablespoon canola oil

5 oz spinach (140 g)

2 cups mushroom (150 g), sliced

1 teaspoon salt

1 teaspoon pepper

1 cup pesto (225 g)

½ cup parmesan cheese (110 g)

½ lb spaghetti (225 g), cooked

Instructions

Heat pot over medium-high heat.

Add oil to the pot.

Cook the spinach until wilted.

Add the mushrooms, salt, and pepper cooking until most of the water is gone.

Add the pesto and parmesan.

Add the spaghetti, and toss until evenly coated, with the sauce sticking to the noodles.

Enjoy!

Caprese Spaghetti Squash

Things Needed

for 2 servings

Squash

1 spaghetti squash

2 tablespoons olive oil

1 teaspoon salt

1 teaspoon pepper

Filling

1 tablespoon oil

3 cloves garlic, minced

½ yellow onion, diced

1 cup cherry tomato (200 g), halved

½ teaspoon salt

½ teaspoon pepper

8 oz mini mozzarella ball (225 g)

fresh basil, to garnish

Instructions

Preheat oven to 400ºF (200ºC).

With a sharp knife, slice the squash in half. If the squash is too tough, puncture in several places forming a dotted line around the squash. Microwave for 3-5 minutes to soften. Allow to cool before cutting in half.

Scoop out the seeds, brush with oil, and sprinkle with salt, and pepper. Bake for 40-45 minutes, or until a fork can easily pierce the skin.

In a pan over medium heat, add the oil, garlic, and onions, and sautè until onions are translucent.

Add the cherry tomatoes, salt, and pepper and simmer until they are cooked and begin to become softened.

Remove squash from the oven, with a fork pull at the edges to produce that stringy "spaghetti" quality. Add the squash to the tomato mixture and mix in the pan.

Add mixture back to the hollowed out spaghetti squash halves. Top with mini mozzarella balls ans basil.

Bake an additional 5-10 minutes, or until cheese melts.

Serve in the squash, and top with basil.

Enjoy!

Crunchy Avocado Tuna Wraps

Things Needed

for 4 servings

5 oz tuna (140 g), 2 cans, drained

1 large avocado, diced

1 cup carrot (110 g), finely chopped

2 ribs celery, finely chopped

¼ cup red onion (35 g), finely chopped

¼ cup dijon mustard (60 g)

1 tablespoon lemon juice

½ teaspoon garlic powder

salt, to taste

pepper, to taste

4 whole wheat tortillas

4 leaves green leaf lettuce

1 cup cherry tomatoes (200 g), halved

Instructions

In a large bowl, add the tuna and avocado. Use a fork to smash the avocado and tuna together.

Add the carrots, celery, red onion, Dijon mustard, lemon juice, garlic powder, salt, and pepper. Stir to combine.

Lay a tortilla flat on a plate. Lay a lettuce leaf on the tortilla. Scoop ¼ of the tuna mixture into the center of the lettuce and spread down the middle. Top with cherry tomatoes and carefully roll the the tortilla to create a wrap. Repeat with the remaining ingredients.

Enjoy!

Tomato Basil Sausage Spaghetti

Things Needed

for 2 servings

½ lb ground sausage (225 g)

½ onion, diced

1 teaspoon salt

1 teaspoon pepper

2 cups marinara sauce (500 g)

1 cup milk (240 mL)

½ cup fresh basil (20 g), chopped

½ lb spaghetti (225 g), cooked

Instructions

Heat pot to medium-high heat.

Cook the sausage in the pot.

Add the onions, salt, and pepper, cooking until the onions are translucent and sausage is starting to brown.

Add the marinara, milk, and basil, cooking until sauce has thickened slightly.

Add the spaghetti, and toss until evenly coated and sauce sticks to the noodles.

Enjoy!

One-Pan Chicken And Broccoli Stir Fry

Things Needed

for 2 servings

1 lb chicken (455 g), cubed

1 teaspoon salt

1 teaspoon pepper

1 cup broccoli (150 g), chopped

1 cup bell pepper (100 g), diced

Stir-Fry Sauce

½ cup soy sauce (120 mL)

¼ cup honey (85 g)

2 cloves garlic

1 teaspoon ginger

1 tablespoon sesame seed

Instructions

Mix together all sauce ingredients in a small bowl.

Heat oil over a nonstick pan and add chicken stirring until cooked.

Pour sauce in pan and stir to coat meat.

Once the sauce is bubbling, add the veggies to the pan and stir again to coat.

Cook until meat is cooked through and veggies are soft.

Serve over rice or alone.

Enjoy!

Slow Cooker Balsamic Chicken

Things Needed

for 4 servings

1 tablespoon olive oil

4 cloves garlic, minced

1 lb baby carrot (455 g)

8 boneless, skinless chicken thighs

1 teaspoon salt

1 teaspoon pepper

1 teaspoon garlic powder

1 teaspoon dried basil

½ cup balsamic vinegar (120 mL)

1 onion, sliced

1 lb green beans (455 g)

fresh parsley, chopped, for garnish

Instructions

Pour olive oil and garlic in the bottom of a 6-qt slow cooker. Line the bottom with baby carrots, then place the chicken thighs over the carrots.

Season the chicken thighs with salt, pepper, garlic powder, basil and vinegar. Top with sliced onion.

Cover and cook on low heat for 8 hours or high for 4 hours. Add green beans during the last 30 minutes of cooking time.

Sprinkle with fresh chopped parsley and serve immediately.

Enjoy!

Instant Pot Butter Chicken

Things Needed

for 4 servings

2 lb boneless, skinless chicken thighs (910 g)

4 teaspoons kosher salt, salt, divided

freshly ground black pepper, to taste

3 tablespoons unsalted butter

1 cup onion (150 g), finely chopped

3 cloves garlic, minced

1 ginger, 2 inch () peeled and minced

2 teaspoons paprika

1 ½ tablespoons garam masala

1 tablespoon curry powder

28 oz crushed tomato (795 g)

1 cup plain whole milk yogurt (245 g)

basmati rice, cooked, for serving

naan bread, for serving

fresh cilantro, for garnish

Instructions

On a cutting board, pat the chicken thighs dry with paper towels. Season chicken on both sides with 1 teaspoon salt and black pepper to taste. Set aside.

Set Instant Pot to high on the sauté setting. Melt the butter in the pot, then add the onion and sauté until it begins to soften, 4 minutes.

Add the garlic and ginger and cook until softened, stirring occasionally, 2 minutes.

Add the remaining 3 teaspoons salt, the paprika, garam masala, and curry powder. Cook, stirring, until the spices are aromatic and toasted, about 1 minute.

Add the crushed tomatoes and the chicken and stir to combine. Place the lid on the Instant Pot and seal to close. Set the machine to pressure cook on high and cook for 5 minutes.

Turn off the Instant Pot and let it vent naturally for 10 minutes. Then turn the quick release seal to "vent" and allow any remaining steam to vent.

Remove the lid. Using tongs, transfer the chicken to a cutting board. When cool enough to handle, cut into bite-sized pieces.

Set the machine to high on the sauté setting. Cook sauce until it is reduced by half, 10–15 minutes.

. Add the yogurt to the sauce and stir to combine. Return the chicken to the pot and stir to coat completely with sauce.

Serve chicken with basmati rice and naan and garnish with cilantro.

Enjoy!

Chickpea Sweet Potato Stew

Things Needed

for 4 servings

2 tablespoons refined coconut oil

1 small onion, diced

3 cloves garlic, minced

1 teaspoon ginger, minced

1 tablespoon sweet paprika

½ teaspoon cumin

¼ teaspoon dried coriander

⅛ teaspoon cayenne

15 oz chickpeas (425 g), 1 can, drained and rinsed

2 cups sweet potato (400 g), peeled and diced

15 oz fire roasted crushed tomato (425 g), 1 can

3 cups vegetable broth (720 mL)

5 oz fresh spinach (140 g)

for 4 servings

2 tablespoons refined coconut oil

1 small onion, diced

3 cloves garlic, minced

1 teaspoon ginger, minced

1 tablespoon sweet paprika

½ teaspoon cumin

¼ teaspoon dried coriander

⅛ teaspoon cayenne

15 oz chickpeas (425 g), 1 can, drained and rinsed

2 cups sweet potato (400 g), peeled and diced

15 oz fire roasted crushed tomato (425 g), 1 can

3 cups vegetable broth (720 mL)

5 oz fresh spinach (140 g)

Instructions

In large pot or Dutch oven, heat the coconut oil over medium heat. Once the oil begins to shimmer, add the onion and cook for 4-5 minutes, or until the onion is semi-translucent.

Add the garlic and ginger, and cook for 2-3 more minutes, until fragrant. Then add the sweet paprika, cumin, coriander, and cayenne and cook for 2 more minutes, until fragrant.

Add the chickpeas, sweet potatoes, crushed tomatoes, and vegetable broth, and bring to a boil. Reduce the heat to medium-low and simmer for 15-20 minutes, or until the sweet potatoes are tender.

Add the spinach and stir until wilted.

Serve immediately.

Enjoy!

Caprese Spaghetti Squash

Things Needed

for 2 servings

Squash

1 spaghetti squash

2 tablespoons olive oil

1 teaspoon salt

1 teaspoon pepper

Filling

1 tablespoon oil

3 cloves garlic, minced

½ yellow onion, diced

1 cup cherry tomato (200 g), halved

½ teaspoon salt

½ teaspoon pepper

8 oz mini mozzarella ball (225 g)

fresh basil, to garnish

Instructions

Preheat oven to 400°F (200°C).

With a sharp knife, slice the squash in half. If the squash is too tough, puncture in several places forming a dotted line around the squash. Microwave for 3-5 minutes to soften. Allow to cool before cutting in half.

Scoop out the seeds, brush with oil, and sprinkle with salt, and pepper. Bake for 40-45 minutes, or until a fork can easily pierce the skin.

In a pan over medium heat, add the oil, garlic, and onions, and sautè until onions are translucent.

Add the cherry tomatoes, salt, and pepper and simmer until they are cooked and begin to become softened.

Remove squash from the oven, with a fork pull at the edges to produce that stringy "spaghetti" quality. Add the squash to the tomato mixture and mix in the pan.

Add mixture back to the hollowed out spaghetti squash halves. Top with mini mozzarella balls ans basil.

Bake an additional 5-10 minutes, or until cheese melts.

Serve in the squash, and top with basil.

Enjoy!

Crunchy Avocado Tuna Wraps

Things Needed

for 4 servings

5 oz tuna (140 g), 2 cans, drained

1 large avocado, diced

1 cup carrot (110 g), finely chopped

2 ribs celery, finely chopped

¼ cup red onion (35 g), finely chopped

¼ cup dijon mustard (60 g)

1 tablespoon lemon juice

½ teaspoon garlic powder

salt, to taste

pepper, to taste

4 whole wheat tortillas

4 leaves green leaf lettuce

1 cup cherry tomatoes (200 g), halved

Instructions

In a large bowl, add the tuna and avocado. Use a fork to smash the avocado and tuna together.

Add the carrots, celery, red onion, Dijon mustard, lemon juice, garlic powder, salt, and pepper. Stir to combine.

Lay a tortilla flat on a plate. Lay a lettuce leaf on the tortilla. Scoop ¼ of the tuna mixture into the center of the lettuce and spread down the middle. Top with cherry tomatoes and carefully roll the the tortilla to create a wrap. Repeat with the remaining ingredients.

Enjoy!

Roasted Eggplant Curry

Things Needed

for 6 servings

3 medium eggplants

¼ cup olive oil (60 mL)

sea salt, to taste

½ teaspoon freshly ground pepper, plus more to taste

¼ cup coconut oil (60 mL)

½ medium white onion, chopped

1 teaspoon chili powder

2 teaspoons ground cardamom

1 teaspoon smoked paprika

1 teaspoon ground coriander

1 tablespoon ground turmeric

3 cloves garlic, minced

1 teaspoon ginger, peeled and minced

3 roma tomatoes, Ripe, Diced, Medium size

15 oz coconut milk (425 mL)

½ cup water (120 mL)

cooked rice, for serving

fresh cilantro, chopped, for serving

Instructions

Preheat the oven to 400°F (200°C).

Slice the tops off the eggplants, then slice them in half lengthwise. Cut each half once more lengthwise. Lay the slices on their flat sides and cut lengthwise into thirds. Finally, slice horizontally to form cubes.

Transfer to a baking sheet, drizzle with the olive oil, salt, and pepper. Bake for 25 minutes, stirring halfway through, until golden brown.

In a large saucepan, heat the coconut oil over high hat. Add the onions, stir for 1 minute, then reduce the heat to medium-low and cook, stirring occasionally, until the onions are golden brown, about 8 minutes.

Stir in the chili powder, cardamom, and smoked paprika. Cook until fragrant, about 1 minute.

Stir in the ground coriander, ½ teaspoon of black pepper, turmeric, garlic, and ginger. Cook for a few minutes more, stirring constantly.

Add the chopped tomatoes, coconut milk, water, and the roasted eggplant.

Bring the curry to a simmer, then reduce to low heat, cover, and simmer for 25 minutes. The sauce should reduce and thicken slightly.

Serve the curry warm over rice, topped with chopped cilantro.

Enjoy!

Parchment Teriyaki Salmon

Things Needed

for 1 serving

½ cup carrot (60 g), thinly sliced

1 cup broccoli floret (250 g)

olive oil, to taste

salt, to taste

pepper, to taste

6 oz skinless salmon (200 g)

2 tablespoons teriyaki sauce

Special Equipment

parchment paper, or aluminum foil, 12×18 inches (30x47cm)

Instructions

Preheat oven to 350°F (180°C).

Fold the parchment paper in half, then open up.

On one half, lay down the broccoli and carrots. Drizzle on oil and sprinkle on salt & pepper.

Lay the salmon on the veggies, and pour on teriyaki sauce.

Fold the parchment paper over the salmon, and cinch the paper together by folding it over itself along the edges.

Bake for 20 minutes or until internal temperature of salmon reaches 145°F (63°C).

Enjoy!

Easy Salmon Dinner

Things Needed

for 2 servings

1 lb potato (455 g)

olive oil, to taste

salt, to taste

pepper, to taste

3 tablespoons lemon juice

2 cloves garlic, minced

½ teaspoon onion powder

½ teaspoon paprika

½ teaspoon dried thyme

½ teaspoon dried parsley

2 tablespoons honey

2 salmon fillets

1 bunch asparagus

6 slices lemon

4 sprigs fresh thyme

Instructions

Preheat oven to 400°F (200°C)

Add potatoes to a parchment paper-lined baking sheet.

Season with olive oil, thyme, salt, and pepper.

Bake for 20 minutes.

To prepare salmon marinade, combine lemon juice, garlic, onion powder, paprika, thyme, parsley, and honey, and stir until evenly combined.

On the same baking tray, push the potatoes to one side of the tray and add salmon and asparagus.

Season the salmon and asparagus with olive oil, salt, and pepper. Brush the marinade on the salmon.

Top salmon with lemon slices and thyme springs.

Bake for 12-14 minutes or until salmon is cooked.

Enjoy!

Sausage, Spinach, Tomato Rigatoni

Things Needed

for 6 servings

1 tablespoon olive oil

5 links hot italian sausage

1 large yellow onion, chopped

5 cloves garlic, minced

salt, to taste

pepper, to taste

1 tablespoon dried oregano

1 tablespoon dried basil

1 tablespoon dried parsley

12 oz tomato paste (340 g)

15 oz diced tomato (425 g)

2 cups grated parmesan cheese (220 g), divided

2 cups spinach (80 g)

1 lb rigatoni (455 g), cooked

1 cup ricotta cheese (245 g)

fresh basil, to garnish

Instructions

To a large dutch oven on medium heat, add the olive oil and heat it until it shimmers.

Add the hot Italian sausage, cook until the the first side browns deeply, flip and cook on the other side until the sausage is fully cooked, 15 minutes. Remove the sausages from the pan and slice when they cool down.

To the leftover pan drippings, add the chopped yellow onion, minced garlic, salt, pepper, dried basil, dried oregano, and dried parsley. Cook until the onions are caramelized and soft. About 10 minutes.

Add the tomato paste and cook until the tomato paste darkens slightly.

Add in the diced tomatoes and the sausage slices into the pan, stir, and let the sauce come to a simmer.

Add in half the grated parmesan, spinach, the cooked pasta, and stir to combine.

Spoon in fresh dollaps of the ricotta cheese, garnish with fresh basil, more grated parmesan, and serve!

Enjoy!

Sesame Peanut Noodles

Things Needed

for 4 servings

½ cup peanut butter (120 g)

3 tablespoons low sodium soy sauce

2 tablespoons sesame oil

2 tablespoons rice vinegar

3 tablespoons water

2 ½ teaspoons brown sugar

1 clove garlic

½ tablespoon fresh ginger, minced

8 oz spaghetti (240 g), cooked according to package instructions

½ cup shredded carrot (55 g)

½ cup shredded red cabbage (50 g)

¾ cup edamame (115 g), shelled

peanut, for garnish

1 tablespoon black sesame seeds, for garnish

scallion, sliced, for garnish

Instructions

In a blender, combine the peanut butter, soy sauce, sesame oil, rice vinegar, water, brown sugar, garlic, and ginger and blend until smooth.

In a large bowl, add the spaghetti, carrots, cabbage, and edamame and pour over the peanut sauce. Use tongs to mix well, until sauce is fully incorporated.

Transfer to bowls and top with peanuts, black sesame seeds, and scallion.

Enjoy!

SWEET TREATS FOR METABOLIC SYNDROME

Strawberry Banana Chia Seed Pudding

Things Needed

for 4 servings

1 banana, mashed

½ cup greek yogurt (140 g)

1 cup almond milk (240 mL)

1 teaspoon vanilla extract

¼ cup chia seeds (40 g)

1 cup strawberry (150 g), diced

Toppings

1 banana, sliced

1 handful strawberry, diced

Instructions

Mash the banana in a medium bowl.

Mix the banana and the yogurt together until smooth.

Pour in the almond milk, vanilla extract, chia seeds, and strawberries, and mix until well combined.

Pour the mixture into an airtight container and refrigerate, covered for 4 hours..

Spoon the pudding into desired serving dish and top with sliced bananas and diced strawberries.

Enjoy!

Easiest Banana-cocoa Ice Cream

Things Needed

for 2 servings

4 bananas

1 tablespoon unsweetened cocoa powder, depending on your taste

¼ teaspoon ground cinnamon

strawberry, to garnish

Instructions

Slice bananas and place in an airtight container. Freeze for at least two hours, preferably overnight.

Place frozen banana slices in a food processor and blend until they reach the consistency of soft serve, about 4 minutes.

Add cocoa powder and cinnamon. Blend until just combined.

Serve immediately for soft-serve consistency or transfer to freezer for at least 2 hours for ice cream consistency.

Garnish with strawberries.

Enjoy!

Strawberry Chocolate Mousse

Things Needed

for 2 servings

6 oz dark chocolate (170 g), 72% is best

½ cup low fat milk (120 mL)

1 teaspoon pure vanilla extract

1 pinch salt

1 cup greek yogurt (285 g)

8 strawberries

Instructions

In a small saucepan, heat milk on medium-low heat until scalding around 180°F (82°C). Do not boil the milk.

Pour hot milk over chocolate.

Add vanilla and salt. Let it stand for 3 minutes to soften.

Whisk together until fully incorporated. Let cool.

Add yogurt. Whisk together until fully incorporated.

Layer chocolate in the bottom of 2 cups followed by strawberries. Repeat until the glasses are full.

Enjoy!

Frozen Banana Ice Cream

Things Needed

for 4 servings

3 ripe bananas

1 tablespoon vanilla extract

¾ cup peanut butter (180 g)

Instructions

Peel the bananas and slice into 1-inch (2 cm) slices.

Spread the bananas on a parchment-lined baking sheet and freeze for 2 hours.

Blend the frozen banana slices in a high-speed blender until they reach a smooth consistency.

Add the vanilla and peanut butter and blend to combine.

Transfer to a bowl or container and freeze for 1 hour, or until ready to serve.

Scoop out ice cream.

Enjoy!

Iced Oatmeal Cookies

Things Needed

for 8 servings

2 cups old fashioned rolled oat (200 g), pulsed in food processor x10

2 cups flour (250 g)

½ teaspoon baking powder

2 teaspoons cinnamon

½ teaspoon nutmeg

1 cup unsalted butter (230 g), room temperature and softened

½ cup sugar (100 g)

1 cup brown sugar (220 g)

1 teaspoon vanilla extract

2 eggs

½ cup raisin (75 g)

Icing

2 cups powdered sugar (220 g)

1 ½ tablespoons milk

1 tablespoon warm water

Instructions

Preheat oven to 350°F (180°C)

Pulse oats in a food processor or blender 10 times.

Add pulsed oats, flour, baking powder, cinnamon, and nutmeg into a bowl.

In a large bowl, beat softened butter with a hand mixer until creamy, add brown and white sugars, then beat until fluffy. Next beat in vanilla and eggs 1 at a time.

Pour the dry Things Needed into the wet ingredients ⅓ at a time until it's gone and dough forms.

Fold in raisins or chocolate chunks.

Take 1 tablespoon of dough and roll it into a ball. Then flatten into a cookie shape and put on a well-greased parchment-lined baking sheet.

Bake 12-15 minutes. (Top rack = no brown bottoms, bottom rack = browned bottoms and a little more crispy).

Cool completely and make the icing in the meantime. Combine powdered sugar, milk, and warm water in a shallow bowl. Once the cookies have cooled, dip into the icing or dab icing on with a pastry brush. Dry for 10 minutes or until icing has hardened.

Enjoy!

Apple Pie (Macerated)

Things Needed

for 8 servings

5 lb granny smith apple (2.2 kg)

1 cup brown sugar (220 g)

¼ teaspoon fine salt

2 teaspoons ground cinnamon

⅓ cup fresh lemon juice (80 mL)

3 ½ tablespoons cornstarch, divided

3 tablespoons water

3 ½ tablespoons unsalted butter

2 premade pie crusts, rolled out into ⅛-inch (3-mm) thick

egg wash

sanding sugar, for sprinkling

Instructions

Peel and thinly slice the apples (keep the apples in a bowl of lemon water as you go to keep them from browning).

In a large bowl, toss the apples with the brown sugar, salt, cinnamon, lemon juice, and half of the cornstarch. Once the apples are well coated, let sit and macerate for 30 minutes, stirring occasionally.

Preheat the oven to 400°F (200°C).

Transfer the apples to a colander set over a medium bowl and let drain for about 15 minutes, until all of the liquid is drawn out.

Transfer the liquid released from the apples to a small pot over low heat.

In a small bowl, mix the rest of the cornstarch and the water to make a slurry. Add the slurry to the apple liquid and quickly stir to incorporate. Bring to a boil, then add the butter and stir until melted. Immediately remove from the heat and pour over the apples, stirring to coat.

Gently lay 1 rolled-out pie crust in a 10-inch (25-cm) pie dish.

Lay the apples in the pie crust, making sure they are flat and facing the rounded edges out in order to fit as many apples as possible in the crust. Pour any leftover liquid from the bowl over the apples.

Top with the other rolled-out pie crust. Trim the excess dough from the edges.

Press the 2 crusts together to seal, then fold the edges under. Crimp the edges.

Then brush all over with egg wash and sprinkle the with sanding sugar.

Use a paring knife to cut a few vents in the top for steam to escape.

Bake for 40-45 minutes, until golden brown.

Let cool for at least an hour

Slice and serve.

Enjoy!

Banana Berry Fruit Salad

Things Needed

for 4 servings

3 bananas, sliced

12 oz fresh strawberry (340 g), quartered

12 oz fresh raspberry (340 g)

Dressing

3 tablespoons lime juice

1 tablespoon maple syrup

Instructions

Combine all the ingredients above in a large bowl.

Mix the dressing ingredients together and spread over fruit, mix well.

Enjoy!

Kiwi Sorbet

Things Needed

for 2 servings

1 lb frozen kiwi (455 g), sliced

¼ cup honey (85 g), or preferred sweetener

Instructions

Blend all Things Needed in a food processor or high-speed blender until thoroughly combined.

Pour into a rectangular loaf pan and smooth into an even layer.

Freeze for 2 hours, or until frozen but still a little soft for scooping. (If freezing overnight, cover with a lid or plastic wrap, but let it sit out at room temperature for about 5-10 minutes before scooping.)

Scoop into a bowl.

Enjoy!

Vegan Apple Pie

Things Needed

for 6 servings

Crust

2 ½ cups all-purpose flour (310 g), plus more for dusting

1 tablespoon organic sugar

1 teaspoon kosher salt

1 cup vegan butter (225 g), cubed and chilled

6 tablespoons ice water

Filling

7 granny smith apples

2 cups organic sugar (400 g), plus 1 teaspoon, divided

1 lemon, zested

5 tablespoons cornstarch

½ lemon, juiced

1 tablespoon coconut oil, melted, plus 1 teaspoon, divided

½ teaspoon salt

4 teaspoons cinnamon, divided

Instructions

Make the crust: In a large bowl, combine the flour, sugar, and salt.

Add the cubed butter, a bit at a time, and use a fork to work it into the flour with a fork until it breaks down to dime-sized pieces.

Gradually add the ice water and mix just until the dough can be pressed together.

Divide the dough in half and shape into discs. Wrap in plastic wrap and chill in the fridge for 1 hour.

Preheat the oven to 350°F (180°C).

Make the filling: Peel and core apples, then thinly slice. Transfer to a large bowl and add 2 cups (200 G) of sugar, the lemon zest, cornstarch, lemon juice, 1 teaspoon melted coconut oil, salt, and 3 teaspoons cinnamon. Toss until the apples are well-coated. Set aside.

On a lightly floured surface, roll out both of the discs of dough to about 1 inch (2 cm) thick. Transfer one round to a greased 8-inch (20-cm) pie dish and gently press against the bottom and sides. Trim the excess dough around the edges, then prick the bottom of the pie crust all over with a fork

Pour the apples into the bottom crust and cover with the top crust. Trim the excess dough around the edges, then crimp the top and bottom crusts together with a fork. Brush the top of the crust with the remaining tablespoon of melted coconut oil and sprinkle with the remaining teaspoon of sugar and cinnamon. Cut 4 vents in the top crust

Bake for 1 hour, until crust is starting to turn golden brown.

Let cool for 10 minutes, then slice and serve.

Enjoy!

Banana Bread Dip

Things Needed

for 4 servings

2 bananas

1 chickpea, 1 can, drained and rinsed

2 tablespoons honey

2 teaspoons vanilla extract

1 teaspoon ground cinnamon

2 tablespoons walnuts, chopped to serve

Instructions

Add bananas, chickpeas, honey, vanilla, and cinnamon to a food processor and blend until smooth.

Top with walnuts and serve with your favorite fruit or dipping snack.

Enjoy!

CHAPTER 6
CONCLUSION

Obesity, hyperlipidemia, insulin resistance, and hypertension are not just isolated health concerns; they are interwoven threads contributing to the intricate tapestry of metabolic syndrome (MetS), a complex constellation of conditions that significantly heightens the risk of cardiovascular diseases. This syndrome, once considered prevalent primarily in affluent, highly urbanized nations like the United States, has now transcended geographical boundaries, spreading its influence to developing nations where rapid urbanization and changes in lifestyle have accelerated its prevalence to alarming epidemic levels.

Within this landscape of metabolic dysfunction, the MetS emerges as a pivotal precursor to a myriad of health complications. Its insidious nature extends beyond the immediate health consequences, permeating various facets of individuals' well-being and societal health burdens. The MetS amplifies the risk of type 2 diabetes by nearly fivefold, casting a shadow of vulnerability over millions worldwide. Moreover, its ominous presence more than triples the likelihood of succumbing to cardiovascular mortality, underscoring the urgency of addressing its multifaceted impacts on global health outcomes.

Delving deeper into the complexities of MetS reveals a web of interconnected physiological pathways and systemic disturbances. While the mechanistic underpinnings of its profound impacts remain shrouded in mystery, emerging evidence suggests that the intricate interplay between metabolic derangements and cardiovascular dysfunction may hold the key to unraveling its enigmatic nature. In particular, the higher mortality rate associated with MetS, even in its nascent stages, raises intriguing questions about the role of the heart's microcirculation as a potential harbinger of cardiovascular injury.

Despite decades of scientific inquiry, the exact mechanisms driving the deleterious effects of MetS continue to elude researchers, presenting an ongoing challenge in the realm of cardiovascular medicine and metabolic health. Thus, the quest for elucidating the intricate pathophysiological pathways underlying MetS remains a pressing imperative, necessitating collaborative efforts across disciplines to untangle the complexities of this pervasive syndrome and pave the way for innovative interventions and targeted therapeutic strategies.

The burgeoning epidemic of metabolic syndrome underscores the critical need for comprehensive preventive measures, early detection strategies, and tailored interventions aimed at mitigating its far-reaching impacts on individual health outcomes and global public health. Only through a concerted, multidisciplinary approach can we hope to navigate the intricate labyrinth of MetS and chart a course towards a healthier, more resilient future for generations to come.